'A compelling account of the trials, tribu[...]
vet – and a lesson to us all on how we sho[...]
we share our lives.'

Stephen Moss, naturalist and author of *The Robin: A Biography*

'Over the years as a vet, I have experienced many of the same situations,
challenges and feelings that Sean reflects on in this incredible book.
He helps us see things from the animals' perspectives, which is one of
the key skills that every vet has to learn. We must, as individuals and as
societies, be responsible for the part we each play in the lives of animals,
whether they be used for food, sport, as our pets or for our enjoyment in
nature. I strongly encourage you to read this book – I believe it helps us to
understand the interwoven challenges we face as we navigate an uncertain
future and equips us with the tools necessary to make a difference. I'm
already telling everyone I know to read it!'

Dr Justine Shotton, President, British Veterinary Association

'Fascinating, engaging, urgent and important. Wensley is the ideal guide
to the mysteries of the animal mind. If this doesn't revolutionize your
view of the food on your plate and the whine of your dog, nothing will.'

Charles Foster, author of *Being a Beast* and *Being a Human*

'*Through a Vet's Eyes* provides a fascinating insight into the lives of
different animals: those that live in the wild, are farmed for human
consumption and the ones we choose to live with in our homes as
domestic pets. The welfare and experiences of the animals who share this
planet with humans in their different ways is told humanely with genuine
compassion that drives home the responsibility we all share to think
about the impact that we have in the way we live our lives.'

**Dr Elaine Mulcahy, Director, UK Health Alliance on
Climate Change**

'Beguiling and devastating, this book explores how to play with a fox and recognize kinship with animals, even as it calmly and kindly reveals the truth of how animals are treated before they are made into food. If you love animals, read this book.'

Jay Griffiths, author of *Wild: An Elemental Journey*

'*Through a Vet's Eyes* is a sensitive and intimate chronicle charting one man's journey through the wonders of the animal and natural world. By blending keen observation and scientific enquiry with an enduring passion for nature, Dr Sean Wensley provides a hugely insightful commentary into our relationship with animals and the wider living environments we co-habit. An excellent read for anyone with an interest in the collective responsibility we all have to ensure the welfare of the animal world and the sustainability and wellbeing of our ecosystems.'

Dr Osman A. Dar, One Health Project Director, Royal Institute of International Affairs, and Working Group Co-chair, One Health High Level Expert Panel (OHHLEP)

'Framed around a compelling and very personal journey, this book is packed with decades of insight. Each chapter dances naturally between nature writing and first-person tales of animals in our care. I loved the storytelling prose, the binocular-clad explorations of a fellow naturalist and the quirky pairings of animals wild and domesticated, all delivered in a tone that is measured yet passionate. And what I really liked is that it's told by a vet, offering the reader fresh perspectives through the eyes of animals.'

Philip Lymbery, CEO, Compassion in World Farming, and author of *Farmageddon: The True Cost of Cheap Meat*

'In this book, Sean Wensley explores some of the ways our human lives are intrinsically linked to those of animals and how a better understanding of these relationships can benefit both. I commend it to anyone who would like to know more about this fascinating subject.'

Dr David Danson, President, Comparative Medicine Section, The Royal Society of Medicine

'An enlightening guide to how scientists get inside the minds of other animals.'
Henry Mance, *Financial Times*

'This deeply thoughtful and insightful book speaks to the heart of our responsibility to animals. Sean Wensley takes off the blinkers, strips away anthropomorphism, and asks us to focus on the species-specific needs of a range of creatures that we may choose to eat, keep as pets, or use in sport or leisure. Utterly humane, evidence-based, and beautifully argued, this book should be read by everyone whose life intersects with those of animals.'
Roly Owers MRCVS, CEO, World Horse Welfare

'A landmark book.'
Marc Bekoff, University of Colorado, author of
The Animals' Agenda

'[*Through a Vet's Eyes*] is comprehensive yet concise, sensitive without being sentimental and idealistic without being overly ideological.
I loved it.'
Josh Loeb, *Vet Record*

'A very good read...I learned a lot. This book should make all of us think more deeply about those animals that are kept for our benefit.'
Mark Avery, environmental campaigner and author of
Remarkable Birds

THROUGH A VET'S EYES

DR SEAN WENSLEY FRCVS

Foreword by Miranda Krestovnikoff, RSPB President

THROUGH A VET'S EYES

How to care for animals and treat them better

First published in Great Britain in 2022 by Gaia, an imprint of
Octopus Publishing Group Ltd
Carmelite House
50 Victoria Embankment
London EC4Y 0DZ
www.octopusbooks.co.uk

An Hachette UK Company
www.hachette.co.uk

ISBN 978-1-85675-475-0

A CIP catalogue record for this book is available from the
British Library.

Printed and bound in the United Kingdom

13 5 7 9 10 8 6 4 2

Some names and descriptions have been changed to protect identities.

Senior Commissioning Editor: Natalie Bradley
Commissioning Editor: Nicola Crane
Senior Editor: Faye Robson
Copy Editor: Sarah Lustig
Art Director: Mel Four
Production Managers: Nic Jones and Lucy Carter

Typesetting: Jeremy Tilson at The Oak Studio Limited

This FSC® label means that materials used for the product have been responsibly sourced

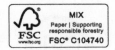

Contents

For Mum, Dad, Jenny, Willow and Enda

'...ABOVE ALL, my constant endeavour will be to ensure the health and welfare of animals committed to my care.'

EXTRACT FROM THE DECLARATION ON ADMISSION TO
THE UK VETERINARY PROFESSION, ROYAL COLLEGE OF
VETERINARY SURGEONS (RCVS), 2012

'We [veterinary surgeons] are clear about our duty to champion animal welfare more broadly across society – beyond the bounds of animals under our direct care – and to challenge activities that compromise animal welfare.' *Vet Futures Report*,
ROYAL COLLEGE OF VETERINARY SURGEONS (RCVS)
AND BRITISH VETERINARY ASSOCIATION (BVA), 2015

'Ensuring good animal welfare is a core mandate of individual veterinarians as well as the veterinary community at large.
It is equally as important to consider and promote positive [animal feelings] as well as to prevent negative ones.'

WORLD VETERINARY ASSOCIATION POLICY ON THE ROLE OF THE
VETERINARIAN IN ANIMAL WELFARE, 2021

Foreword

Miranda Krestovnikoff

Eight years ago, my husband and I sat down at the kitchen table with Sean for his advice. We were thinking about getting a puppy. Carefully, meticulously and unemotionally, Sean talked us through the process, asking us all the right questions to find out why we thought it was a good idea, how it would affect our family life and whether we could give her the care and attention that she needed. Today, we are going through that same process once more, without him beside us, but at every turn we ask ourselves: 'What would Sean do?' His wise words, sound advice and genuine concern about our welfare as well as hers are at the forefront of our minds as we embark on this massive decision once more. She's arriving tomorrow...and the adventure begins!

I've never really had the chance to formally thank Sean for the inspiration he has been to me and to my family, so I'm taking the opportunity to do it here. For my children, he was just 'always there' – another member of the family, but a fairly unusual one, who revived a grass carp, performed post-mortems of our old laying chickens and pointed out the 'copulating kestrels' in the poplar trees ('Mummy, what's "copulating"?' came the reply from my youngest). Sean was our lodger for nearly five years. Apparently, he knew we were the right family to live with after spotting a copy of *BBC Wildlife* magazine on the kitchen table. I imagine that the bird feeders and large wildlife pond also gave away our family's passion for attracting nature into our garden.

Sean introduced us to so many sights and sounds in our garden and beyond. A keen birdwatcher, he could correctly identify a species from a mere fluttering in the bushes, when all I could see was an LBJ ('little brown job'). It took a while for us to realize that he was colour blind, as he could describe birds in such detail that you had no idea that several colours were indistinguishable to him, compared to the kaleidoscope that we experienced from our feathered garden visitors. We have fond memories of a myriad of wildlife experiences with him, such as his spotting a black redstart (my first), which got some of our local twitchers very excited!

Perhaps what we are most grateful for is that Sean pointed out kestrels flying and hunting over the fields that surround our house and, knowing our interest in the local buzzard population, tentatively suggested we could encourage these raptors to the edge of our garden by building and erecting a kestrel box. There then ensued a great deal of research into boxes, materials and construction, and the suitable dwelling was created. Because of Sean, our lives are now intrinsically linked with these birds, as they have nested every subsequent year and we delight in hearing their calls as we leave the house in the morning. We eagerly anticipate the time of fledging when we can watch the acrobatics and mastery of skills as the adults teach their chicks to hunt and to fend for themselves.

Being long-time owners of laying chickens, as well as various pets that the children have grown up with, having a vet and an expert on animal welfare living with us certainly sparked some interesting conversations concerning the animals that we share our lives with. Do the chickens have enough space in their pen in the garden? Are they warm enough overnight? Is the electric fence working? Are the older, non-layers OK? I'm not sure if the stick insects' welfare was ever discussed but I remember that when considering purchasing guinea pigs for the children, and further down the line our puppy, he was always there to offer advice: never judgemental and always impartial, with just a flavour of what he would recommend. In the end, he made it very clear – here is the information, but the choice is, ultimately, up to you.

While he was living with us, Sean talked about a book he had long wanted to write. Given that he has lived a life devoted to improving the welfare of pet, farm and wild animals, I believe Sean is the only person who could have written a book like this. His thoughtful and deeply caring nature comes across in the way he deals with each topic, combining his extensive experience in the field with detailed research and consultations with experts in each and every chapter. Added to that, writing had to be put on hold for a while as he took on the prestigious role of British Veterinary Association officer, becoming the (then) youngest ever President of BVA – one of his many and ever-accumulating accolades.

I am delighted that he has chosen not just to write about animal welfare and ethics, but also to intertwine this with stories about his passion for wildlife. It takes the reader deeply and intimately into Sean's life as a naturalist. I feel as though I have a better insight into and understanding of how deeply rooted is his connection with nature and how intensely he cares about animals by being immersed into some of the wildlife-watching experiences he shares.

As humans, our lives are so intrinsically linked with the creatures that share them it's a wonder that we are so disconnected from the hidden misery and suffering animals endure for our growing consumption and entertainment. In our homes, most of us strive to make our pets' lives as comfortable, interesting and stress-free as possible, so why do other animals deserve any less? These are complicated questions, discussed with consideration and moderation. Sean shares valuable information in these pages, empowering consumers to drive change through what we buy and the choices we make. It is a reminder that we are all able to make changes that will have long-lasting repercussions for the lives and well-being of the animals we come into contact with every day. There is a moral requirement for them to live well and we all have the ability to help to make that happen.

Miranda Krestovnikoff
President of the Royal Society for the Protection of Birds (RSPB)
2021

CHAPTER 1

Beneath the skin

Another anatomy class finished. I leave the echoey confines of the dissection room, along the corridors of skeletons and specimens, and heave my might against the weighty veterinary faculty doors. The university's majestic Victoria Building throws a gothic clock tower high into the Liverpool skyline. I crane at its base, peering upwards at spires that point to a blue sky beyond. Behind me, buses and taxis rumble upon a busy road.

A shrill 'kee kee kee' forks through the urban din: a sound from the wild. I stop dead and look up. A pair of kestrels soar on outstretched wings. Wheeling in interlocking circles, one gathers speed, propelling towards the other, who inverts and the couple lock talons. A courting pair or territorial defence; love or war in the city sky.

The railway from Liverpool to Southport transects the human landscape, passing from inner city to suburbs to areas of open country-side. Trundling above the dark-brick terraces while passengers look in to backyards below, I see dogs pacing and rabbits in small hutches, corrugated roofs and barbed wire. Running parallel to the Mersey, the

1

train continues on until light begins to breathe between the buildings and wild shrubbery bursts from every available gap, beyond suppression. Playing fields – often dusted with wild geese and wading birds in winter mists – and then come the first glimpses of the Sefton coastal dune system. Like a great geographical accordion, the bellows are now fully expanded, roaring with leaves, grasses, limitless horizons, insects, birds, sneaked glimpses, suffocating spectacles: the stuff of wild air. But the journey is dipping in and out of suburbia – these tastes of the wild spaces are like intermittent consciousness in a narcotic dream. By the time I reach my stop, I am among gardens and tree-lined roads.

It has been a long day studying, and I drop my backpack at home and pull on some outdoor trousers and boots. The pockets are like old friends, waiting to receive unusual shells, nibbled pinecones, the day's natural curios. I set off back towards the railway station and, after just five minutes, have crossed the railway line through a metal gate offering quiet support from a mental health charity's posters and am on a dusty track – Fisherman's Path. It crosses the manicured green swathe of Formby golf links, then enters the dark, foreboding cathedral of the coast's pinewoods. It is quiet beneath the towering trees but for the faint, high-pitched contact calls of dainty goldcrests and coal tits. I stop still and hear tiny glass baubles breaking in the branches, each releasing their drops of pine oil, which permeate through the plantation on the sea breeze.

The coniferous woods open out to brighter alder woods whose roots find their essential water in the dune slacks. In a matter of paces, the track turns to sand. My boots push down, sinking into the soft sand as my heart surges forward with each step. As I trudge higher, the hardened coastal shrubs give way to marram grass, swaying comfortably, perfectly adapted to this unforgiving boundary between land and salted gales. When I have climbed high enough, the rolling sea and the dipping sun behind it are so perfect, so welcome, so overwhelming that, as always, it causes me to gasp and grips me so tightly that I must catch my breath. There is warm air on my face. I walk with renewed determination across the dimpled plateau, jump two-footed into a depression on the other side and take large strides down towards the shore. It is evening and this path emerges at a quiet part of the beach; there is nothing but open space in all directions and no one but me.

This part of the Irish Sea is invariably calm and still, though violent storms can eat the dunes with vicious bites. Grey seals bob offshore in the summer months and bright white gannets fly further out, but I can see neither this evening.

My mind is uncluttered. This is home: the most real place on earth. The runnels in the sand reflect the light from the closing day, wrapping me in streaked clouds. The beach stretches as far as I can see, to my left and to my right. It meets a sea that covers all the earthbound space behind me, straining to the shore, and a sky that sweeps above. It is a colossal swirling continuum of sand, sea and sky, timeless and wild. I am absolutely nothing: another grain of sand, flailing matter on the strandline. If I spread my arms and legs as far and wide as I can, then pick apart each of my thoughts and emotions, and pull them as far as they will unravel in all directions – all I have ever known and all I will ever know – I am still absolutely nothing. In this timeless wild landscape, I am just me. This is the purest beauty I know.

Today's anatomy demonstrator was Dr Bajaj, known and respected for his soft, machine-gun fire of precise anatomical terms. He focussed intently on the dog beneath his fingers and scalpel, and quietly directed streams of terminology into the moist spaces created by his prying and cutting. We strained towards video monitors and speakers to concentrate on his quiet, learned output. After about ten minutes, he dismounted from his podium to ensure we had all found for ourselves the structures that he had so nimbly revealed, with our resulting embarrassment if the focus of the day's lesson had accidentally been chopped in half.

In dissection classes, I was fascinated by foramina. Foramen (plural, foramina) is Latin for 'hole', and anyone who has held and inspected a bone will know that their surfaces are pitted and punctured by depressions and small holes. These, perhaps, are not fascinating in themselves, until it is revealed that the porosity of our osseous framework – and that of the rest of the animal kingdom – is not random, but structured purposefully and consistently to enable a precise function: that of providing protective bony tunnels through which frail nerves and blood vessels can pass. What look like random holes dotted around the surface of any given bone are, in fact, part of the precise architecture of living creatures.

Bones, like any other living tissue, need a blood supply. Where arteries that supply nutrients to bones emerge from holes on a bone's surface, the holes are called 'nutrient foramina'. Nutrient foramina exist right across the animal kingdom, within the bones of mammals and birds, reptiles and amphibians. Other foramina are the exit points for nerves.

It is important for trainee medical professionals, such as veterinarians (vets), doctors and dentists, to be aware of foramina because, on an X-ray, a nutrient foramen could be mistaken for a subtle fracture if the practitioner is not au fait with normal anatomy. Foramina that house nerves also need to be learned so that, if necessary, nerve 'blocks' can be applied to provide local anaesthesia. This involves injecting local anaesthetic around a nerve as it emerges from a bony foramen, numbing the surrounding area so that surgical procedures can be performed painlessly.

What fascinated me was the 'sameness' in the bony architecture of all the mammals that we dissected. The more comparative anatomy that we studied – comparing different species that came beneath our scalpels – the more the realization dawned just how similar all mammals are, right down to the level of their foramina.

Flicking through the pages of a veterinary or medical anatomy textbook quickly reveals that the infraorbital foramen, for example, is present in dogs, cats, cattle, horses and humans: in fact, just about any mammal one cares to mention. The same hole, at the same relative position, carrying the same nerve.

There are many larger, more obvious structures we could choose to illustrate the anatomical similarities between mammals. What about the bones, of which foramina are just a part? All mammals have similar limb bones, for example, all arranged in the same order.

Take a human arm first. Starting at the top, we have the shoulder blade, or scapula. Then the humerus. Then the radius and ulna. Then the metacarpals. Then the digits – our fingers – five of them.

What about a dog? At the top, scapula. Then the humerus. Then radius and ulna. Then metacarpals. Then the digits – five of them (one, the so-called dewclaw, is up round the side).

How about a creature that seems more different: a seal? Dissect a seal's flipper and, sure enough, we find scapula, followed by humerus, followed by radius and ulna, followed by digits – five of them.

This pattern of bones in mammals is called the 'pentadactyl limb'.

Pentadactyl literally means 'five digits'. In some mammals, such as cattle and horses, the number of functional digits has reduced (cattle, for example, have dewclaws, like dogs), but the basic underlying pattern is the same.

One of the first, and most famous, scientists to write about the extraordinary anatomical similarities between mammals was Charles Darwin:

> What can be more curious than that the hand of a man, formed for grasping, that of a mole for digging, the leg of the horse, the paddle of the porpoise, and the wing of the bat, should all be constructed on the same pattern, and should include similar bones, in the same relative positions?

Anatomical sameness exists throughout the mammalian body. If we lay a dead human, dog, lion and rat on their backs and peel back their chests and abdominal walls to expose their internal organs, we find the same organs, in the same relative positions, lying beneath – heart, lungs, liver, stomach, spleen, kidneys, intestines, bladder, etc. And, perhaps even more remarkably, these structures are not just anatomically similar, but functionally similar as well. The four-chambered heart of a pig, human, horse or dog – just about any mammal – is, in life, pumping blood around the bodies of each in exactly the same way.

Even at the cellular level – the level of the microscopic cells that are the building blocks of tissues and organs, far smaller than the foramina that caught my attention – we find that cells of a particular type are broadly similar across all species.

The study of cells and tissue at the microscopic level is called histology. At vet school, many students, including myself, used the colourful textbook *Wheater's Functional Histology: A Text and Colour Atlas*. Why is this noteworthy? Because the vast majority of images used in Wheater's textbook, taken using a photomicroscope, are of human tissues. And yet, as the book's preface explains, 'this book should adequately encompass the requirements of undergraduate courses in medicine, dentistry, veterinary science, pharmacy, mammalian biology and allied fields'. It is fine for a veterinary student to use a human histology textbook, because a liver cell is histologically a liver cell, regardless of mammalian species!

Upon learning that I am a vet, people often graciously comment how challenging my work must be 'with so many different types of animals to learn and know about'. I try to reply with humility, but really I, and my colleagues, bask in false glory if people do not realize just how similar – anatomically and functionally – one mammal is from the next. Of course there are species differences in, for example, parasite and pathogen susceptibility, pharmacological considerations and nutritional requirements, but there is also much overlap. Vets, doctors and dentists all essentially practise 'mammal medicine', with vets throwing in – to a greater or lesser extent – reptiles, birds, amphibians and invertebrates for good measure.

Even when it comes to medicine and surgery, there is much overlap between humans and non-human mammals in the fundamental principles. Numerous comments made during medical conversations with friends and acquaintances make me suspicious that people rarely have cause to reflect on how similar humans are to other mammals.

I was introduced to an optometrist, who spoke of a diagnostic dye applied to the eyes of her human patients to detect corneal damage. I enquired if this was fluorescein dye. 'Yes...' she answered, 'how do you know? Do you use it in animals?'

She seemed surprised that this might be the case. But why, when one considers that the cornea is not a human structure, but a structure common to mammals, birds and reptiles, with fluorescein dye used diagnostically in all three?

In a similar case, another non-veterinary acquaintance was telling me about her diagnosed spinal troubles. There is much overlap between medical and veterinary medical terminology, and my apparent familiarity with the basics led her to ask, again with surprise, 'So do animals suffer from disc troubles as well?' In my head, bells were ringing: 'Yes! Of course they do! Why wouldn't they?! They have almost the same vertebral structures, and similar things can go wrong! A slipped disc is as troublesome for a dachshund (a commonly afflicted dog breed) as it is for a person!'

Yet we seem to find it hard to comprehend the sameness between humans and non-human animals.

So what is the point in this fascination with inter-species sameness? It is because understanding the fundamental anatomical and functional similarities between humans and other animals takes us to the heart of why we must extend our circle of compassion to include non-human animals.

We advocate fair and just treatment for all humans, regardless of, for example, age, sex or ethnicity, based on our common capacities for pleasure and pain, and there being things that matter to us all. Based on these same principles, we could expect that all mammals would justifiably argue for their fair and just treatment, if they were offered the language that enabled them to do so.

But does this – the idea of language, and other such capabilities often considered to be uniquely human – bring us to the stumbling block, the fatal flaw in this line of reasoning? We may accept all that has been said thus far about cross-species similarity, but at the end of the day a human is not a dog, a rat, a hedgehog, a whale or a deer. They all seem so different.

This is the crux. If we are to devote our attention, in later chapters, to the beauty of the natural world and the injustices to which we subject our fellow creatures, then we should pursue our concept of mammalian sameness into the brain. Concern for the wellbeing of non-human animals is pointless and misplaced if those animals are not sentient: that is, having the capacity to feel things and to be able to consciously experience feelings that matter to them, such as pain, fear, comfort and enjoyment. If we share the rest of our organs with the other six thousand or so mammalian species, do we also share similar brains?

Superficially, at the gross, dissectible level, most mammalian brains do, indeed, look remarkably similar. To view this for yourself, visit the online mammalian brain museum at www.neurosciencelibrary.org and click on 'List of specimens', where you will find hundreds of clearly labelled photographs. This is what we would expect – why would all our other organs look largely similar, but not our brains?

Physical sameness is present, but what about functional sameness? The brain has a tiered structure; let's say, in mammals, a cauliflower (comprising a stalk surrounded by florets) perched upon a parsnip, which is joined to a courgette. It is the highly folded cauliflower that most people think of if they are asked to picture a brain.

The spinal cord, transmitting information to and from the rest of the body, enters the brain at the courgette. Information then passes through the parsnip, through the cauliflower stalk and on up to the cauliflower florets. Although there are various interconnections between them, each of the constituent parts (each vegetable, if you like) has its own functional responsibilities.

The courgette, parsnip and cauliflower stalk are present in reptiles, birds and mammals, and their functions are essentially the same across all three groups.

Only when we come to the cauliflower florets do significant differences start to appear; extras start to be added in. Language, complex emotions and self-awareness are features of the advanced cauliflower. As you might have guessed, it is mammals like humans and great apes (such as chimpanzees and gorillas) who have advanced cauliflowers.

But what comes with the standard brain model – the basic courgette, parsnip and cauliflower stalk? Remember it is all mammals, birds and reptiles who have these fitted as standard.

The courgette represents the part of the brain called the 'medulla oblongata', often referred to as simply the 'medulla'. This controls fundamental life functions such as breathing, swallowing and heart rate.

The parsnip represents the part of the brain known as the 'midbrain'. This deals with visual and auditory information.

The cauliflower stalk represents structures such as the thalamus, hypothalamus and amygdala. The thalamus plays an important role in regulating sleep and wakefulness; the hypothalamus controls a number of body functions, including thermoregulation (responding to heat and cold), hunger and thirst; the amygdala is associated with fear and anxiety.

Finally, the cauliflower florets represent the cerebrum, and its folded outer layer the cerebral cortex, which is associated with intelligence, learning, memory and language. It should make perfect sense that some animals should have more florets than others (representing greater folding), based on the intuitive observation that some animals seem more 'clever' than others.

But before we get caught up with cleverness, just take a moment to think back to what we've passed on the way to the cauliflower florets – parts of the brain, conserved across reptiles, birds and mammals, capable of generating feelings such as fear, hunger and thirst, and the feelings of being too hot or too cold. Pain mechanisms, too, are highly similar between humans and other animals, with pathways responsible for pain passing through many of the areas we have visited, such as the medulla, midbrain, thalamus and cerebrum.

Reducing something as complex as a brain to a series of three vegetables is, needless to say, a gross oversimplification, but for the purpose of our question it covers the relevant bases. Are the brains of non-human animals functionally similar to those of humans and capable of generating pain, suffering and other feelings? The neuroanatomical and neurophysiological evidence suggests that the answer is yes. Important ingredients of possible suffering, such as pain, hunger and fear, are all considered to be generated by similar brain areas present in animals and humans. Taken to this level – to the very brain itself – the notion of human–animal sameness has crucial implications for how, morally, we should respect and treat the animals from whom we gain so much.

Let's be clear about what brain studies do not tell us. They do not, for example, tell us definitively what animals are capable of experiencing. But this is equally true for fellow people.

A neighbour may tell me that he is scared. He may be frozen to the spot, trembling, pale, wide-eyed and sweating, and if I were to scan his brain, the regions associated with fear might be lit like beacons. But I will never know, for certain, what it is like for that man to experience fear, because I will never be able to enter his private mental world.

But practically, of course, I think I know perfectly well how his fear feels. After all, he is a human male, like me, and when I am afraid I also tremble, become pale, wide-eyed and sweat, and the same fear regions of my brain also light up on scans.

By now you will be well-versed in the reasoning that follows – what about when a horse (or mouse, or sea lion, or sheep, or...) is faced by something they are apparently scared of? When they freeze, tremble, become wide-eyed, and the fear regions from scans of their brain – that we know is anatomically and functionally similar to ours – beam out like beacons? We don't know, for certain, what fear feels like for a horse, but the behavioural, physiological and neurobiological evidence suggesting that it is highly comparable to the human experience is compelling.

It should probably come as little surprise that basic (but important) feelings such as pain, hunger and fear should be so conserved across animal species, being, as they are, crucial for survival. An animal who did not feel hunger would die from starvation, and those who did not experience, and respond to, a 'healthy' fear would fall victim to any of a multitude of dangers present in a natural environment. But what about so-called 'higher' feelings that are generated at the level of the cauliflower florets, the cerebrum? Are these shared by human and non-human animals as well?

Brain-imaging studies of guinea pigs have shown that when they are separated from their young, the part of their brain that is activated is the same as in humans who are experiencing grief. Similarly, if a ewe is viewing her lamb, or an attractive ram, the brain activity seen on scans is fundamentally similar to that seen when humans are shown pictures of their children, or of a romantic partner. Findings such as these do little to refute the argument that the mental lives of animals and humans may bear striking similarities on several important levels.

Let's briefly return to cleverness. Probably the greatest barrier that prevents people from allowing themselves to believe that animals and humans might share a common subjective world is the vast chasm that seemingly exists between human and animal intelligence. 'If animals shared our brain capabilities, then surely we would find otters writing symphonies and meerkats labouring to build space stations?' people sometimes proffer, sarcastically. The route to approaching this has already been mapped out. It may be true that otters, meerkats and most, if not all, other animals, are not as clever as humans (at least, by our typical measures – some mammals and birds outperform people on memory tasks and all animals are as clever as they need to be), but is this at all relevant to whether or not we should treat them humanely? The bottom line is this: animals do not have to be clever to suffer, or to enjoy life. Farmed animals may look stupid slopping around in their own slurry while vacantly chewing their cud (we will see in later chapters that, in fact, commonly farmed animals are far from stupid), but this is irrelevant to the question of whether or not they can experience pain, fear, comfort and pleasure.

In terms of advanced cauliflowers (remember, these are present in those we perceive as the most intelligent mammals, such as humans, great apes and dolphins), it is actually difficult to say with certainty what effect they have on the quality of the lives of animals who carry them. One ability of clever animals, such as great apes, is that they may have a 'theory of mind'; they act as if they can 'think about thinking'. Animals with a theory of mind (like humans) are believed to be able to reflect on their own thoughts and think about the mental states of others. This is an advanced mental ability and it raises the concern that in, for example, animal research laboratories, a particularly intelligent animal, like a chimpanzee, could think about him- or herself in a particular situation in the future and suffer dread about what might happen. They could also suffer from the knowledge that a brother, sister or friend may be in pain.

Alternatively, it has been suggested that some aspects of the suffering of clever animals might be less, because they can rationalize, based on previous experience, that the pain, or some other negative experience, will go away. A 'simpler' animal, however, may not be able to cope in this way, instead just feeling terrible and having no idea when the feeling will stop.

Consideration of sameness should not be restricted to mammals. We have noted, on several occasions, that some of the most fundamental ingredients of suffering – pain, fear, hunger and thirst – are common to reptiles, birds and mammals. The brains of birds and reptiles do not so visibly resemble human brains in the way that those of other mammals do, but both birds and reptiles have brain regions that share similarities with the cerebral cortex (the outer brain layer that deals with our 'higher' functions, such as learning abilities). The derogatory term 'bird brain', used to describe someone supposed to have limited intellectual abilities, is misguided. On reptiles, Professors Anna Wilkinson and Oliver Burman and their colleagues are making fascinating and morally relevant discoveries at the University of Lincoln's Cold-Blooded Cognition Lab, including the abilities of reptiles to demonstrate complex social learning and extensive long-term memory.

In *Hugh's Chicken Run* – a television programme in which British celebrity chef Hugh Fearnley-Whittingstall highlighted animal welfare problems associated with commercial poultry farming – residents of a British town were charged with the task of rearing some chickens for eventual killing and eating. One participant noticed that the chickens followed him when he turned the soil with a pitchfork, so that they might consume any revealed invertebrates (as robins follow gardeners and clouds of white gulls follow the plough). He exclaimed, 'I'm sure they are intelligent! Y'know, they've got a memory. Why are they following me, like this? They know there's something good on the end of the fork, surely!'

Perhaps it's the huge numbers in which we farm some animals – faceless, personality-devoid masses – that cause us to eventually view them as mindless robots. But chickens, like most birds, are eminently capable of learning and display signs of empathy. In fact, the mental abilities of some birds (like crows and parrots) have been found to parallel those of apes. This said, we must not forget the golden rule: an animal does not have to be clever to suffer.

In light of such findings, in 2012 a prominent international group of cognitive neuroscientists, neuropharmacologists, neurophysiologists, neuroanatomists and computational neuroscientists gathered at Cambridge University to discuss animal consciousness and made the

Cambridge Declaration on Consciousness:

> The weight of evidence indicates that humans are not unique in possessing the neurological substrates that generate consciousness. Nonhuman animals, including all mammals and birds, and many other creatures, including octopuses, also possess these neurological substrates.

In some parts of the world, animal sentience is recognized in legislation. In the European Union, the 2007 Lisbon Treaty stipulates that, as sentient beings, full regard should be paid to animals' welfare requirements. Having left the European Union, the UK government announced a new Animal Welfare (Sentience) Bill in 2021, to put 'animal welfare at the very heart of government policy decision making'. The campaign group Crustacean Compassion, backed by, among others, the British Veterinary Association – the national representative body for veterinarians in the UK – successfully lobbied to ensure the provisions of this Bill include decapod crustaceans such as crabs and lobsters, and cephalopod molluscs such as octopus. An independent review published in November 2021 concluded there is strong scientific evidence for the sentience of these animals, who are subjected to practices such as being shrink-wrapped and boiled while alive.

Charles Darwin recognized the pentadactyl limb as representing some of the strongest evidence for the theory of evolution. Verlyn Klinkenborg wrote that Darwin showed humans 'their true ancestry in nature'. Few truer words could be spoken. When our common ancestry with the rest of the natural world is comprehended, it is on at least two levels. First, the ecological level: the level on which humans and all other species on the planet are interconnected in a great, beautiful, interdependent web of life. And second, the common ancestry level: in this, together with all other animal species, we are constructed of the same building blocks and share common structures with common functions. At the level of the brain, we share our pleasure and pain.

Issues involving animals can be highly emotive. Be they the hunting of foxes or the long-distance transport of farmed animals, outpourings of angry, pleading and desperate human emotion can sweep a nation. Humans have debated for millennia how we ought to treat non-human animals: Pythagoras, for example, now better remembered for his mathematics, promoted the ethical treatment of animals, as did 19th-century Romantics such as William Blake ('A Robin Red breast in a Cage/ Puts all Heaven in a Rage'). But such concern, bubbling through our history, lacked a certain something. While it could be tackled by the great minds of the day, with intellectual rigour and within the boundaries of carefully constructed ethical frameworks, it still fundamentally sought to address a seemingly intractable problem. To be concerned for the welfare of animals is to be concerned with the private, inaccessible, mental experiences of species that might be quite unlike us.

Anthropomorphism is the projection of human emotions and motivations onto inanimate objects, natural phenomena or animals, and some have dismissed concern for the proper treatment of animals as anthropomorphic: pursued by 'bunny-huggers' and peddlers of soppiness, sentiment and misplaced emotion. But today, in the 21st century, and uniquely in our history, such a view is especially unenlightened. Since the latter part of the previous century, and continuing now, scientific objectivity has been brought to questions about animal minds and experiences – such as the brain-imaging studies already mentioned – with results that are forcing us to revisit and re-evaluate our ethical debates and positions. Animal welfare, a subject intricately linked with animal feelings and human values, now has science shining into all of its corners. As for most fields, the beam is, in some places, insufficiently bright, but questions about how animals perceive the world, how they think and feel, and what makes them feel good and bad, are now firmly in the hands of scientific inquiry.

The eminent animal welfare lawyer Dr Mike Radford summarizes why animal welfare science has been so influential:

1. Science has an international perspective; its findings are applicable throughout the world.
2. Politicians (and judges) are more likely to adapt their decisions in the light of scientific evidence on the basis that it rises above mere emotion.
3. The insight into the needs and experiences of animals that has been gained through research has had a profound effect on the ethical debate about our relationship with other species and the manner in which we keep them.

The stimulus for this historically unique era of scientific inquiry is largely attributed to a British author, Ruth Harrison. After the Second World War, animal agriculture had become highly mechanized and industrialized, and in her book *Animal Machines*, published in 1964, Harrison revealed the barren and behaviourally restrictive conditions in which so-called 'factory-farmed' animals were being reared. The book stirred intense reaction among the British public and, in response, the government of the day appointed a committee, under the chairmanship of Professor F W Rogers Brambell, to investigate 'the welfare of animals kept under intensive livestock husbandry systems'. The committee, comprising several scientists as well as agriculturalists, made recommendations on various animal husbandry systems, but additionally called for research in fields including veterinary science, stress physiology and animal behaviour to help answer the questions that had arisen about animal farming. Such research began in earnest and gave rise to the field now known as animal welfare science.

Due to the high level of confinement that characterized factory farming, the report of the Brambell Committee concluded that animals should have the freedom to 'stand up, lie down, turn around, groom themselves and stretch their limbs', a list that became known as 'Brambell's Five Freedoms'. Such a list represented substantial progress at the time, but by focussing entirely on physical possibilities it failed to capture other elements of an animal's welfare, which subsequent analysts considered to be important. Welfare, or wellbeing, as we know from our own experience, is a conglomerate concept. That is to say, our wellbeing at any given time is determined by several contributing factors, many of which interact with each other. Our wellbeing is diminished if we have a satisfying and nutritious, balanced diet, but go home to a house that is intolerably hot or cold. We may be in peak physical fitness with access to the highest standards of medical care but endure chronic loneliness. Welfare depends on more than one determinant. By re-examining the original Five Freedoms, the internationally renowned Professor Emeritus of animal welfare John Webster, as a member of the UK-based Farm Animal Welfare Council (FAWC, an independent advisory council to the UK government – now, with a broader remit, called the Animal Welfare Committee), proposed a more comprehensive framework, incorporating both physical health and mental wellbeing. The resulting Five Freedoms have since been used to assess the welfare of animals by governments and non-governmental organizations around the world:

1. freedom from hunger and thirst
2. freedom from discomfort
3. freedom from pain, injury or disease
4. freedom to express normal behaviour
5. freedom from fear and distress.

John Webster himself acknowledged that not all of the Five Freedoms will be met all of the time, while more recent work by FAWC and others has emphasized the importance of providing positive experiences for animals, rather than simply aspiring to freedom from the worst. Nevertheless, the Five Freedoms (and related frameworks, such as the Five Domains, which put additional important emphasis on animals' mental states) can help map a route to a state of animal welfare that incorporates most, if not all, relevant determinants.

The Animal Welfare Acts of 2006 and the Welfare of Animals Act of 2011 in Northern Ireland translated the Five Freedoms into updated UK animal welfare legislation. Each Act introduced a legal duty requiring that a person responsible for an animal's welfare meets the animal's following five needs:

1. the need for a suitable environment
2. the need for a suitable diet
3. the need to be able to exhibit normal behaviour patterns
4. the need to be housed with, or apart from, other animals
5. the need to be protected from pain, suffering, injury and disease.

These so-called Five Welfare Needs have moved the Five Freedoms concept from a theoretical aspiration to a legal obligation in the UK.

How, ethically, can we act on our understanding that many animals that we currently use for our benefit are sentient? Broadly, in one of two ways. We may take an animal rights view, concluding that their similarities to people are grounds for them being granted similar rights – for example, to not be killed for food, enslaved as pets or objectified for our entertainment. In this view, recognition of animal sentience should result in abstention – sentient animals are not ours to use. Or we may take an animal welfare-based view, in which we deem it acceptable to use sentient animals for our benefit (as companions, for food, for sport and so on), as long as, in return, they are afforded a good life and a humane death. In practical terms, their Five Welfare Needs should be met, resulting in good physical health and mental wellbeing; they should be given opportunities to enjoy their lives; and their death should not be associated with preventable pain and suffering.

As a veterinary surgeon – first practising and latterly developing veterinary animal welfare policy with species-specialist colleagues – and during my five years as a veterinary student, I have been privileged to have had first-hand exposure to many of the ways in which animals are used by humans today. In doing so, I have become aware of how billions of animals are not having their Five Welfare Needs met; those cases where we are not meeting our side of the ethical bargain that we strike with sentient animals. It is my professional responsibility to advocate for these animals' best interests, both within the bounds of the status quo (how we currently use animals) and to challenge the status quo (asking, how should we use animals?)

Like many people, I tend to take an animal welfare-based view of how we should use animals. But, within that, I am comfortable that if animals are routinely failing to have their welfare needs met under a certain type of activity (for example as pets or on farms) and this cannot be rectified, then ongoing societal acceptance of that activity will, and should, diminish.

Animal-using activities are woven through our human societies around the world. Pets give companionship and enjoyment; many people eat meat and dairy products; we take medicines that have been tested on animals; some people wear clothing made from animals; and some enjoy animal-based sporting and cultural events. Each of us has an animal welfare footprint, akin to a carbon footprint, the size of which is linked to our everyday decisions and purchases. In this book, I look at some of the welfare problems experienced by animals used for three purposes – for food, for entertainment and as our companions – together with wild animals impacted by human activities. To describe these problems is not to irresponsibly criticize, it is to help us, as societies, understand and account for the ethical costs of these activities, to guide our future choices.

Several chapters are focussed on animals farmed for food. Principally, this is because of the numbers of animals involved and the potential for large-scale animal suffering; over a billion are reared for food every year in the UK, excluding many millions of farmed fish, and over

70 billion globally. In the time it takes to read a page of this book, around 2,000 chickens will have been killed to eat in the UK and 18,000 in the United States.

It is also a critical time for global animal agriculture. Questions of animal welfare on the world's farms are intimately connected with other pressing issues, including climate change, biodiversity loss, human health and accessible, affordable food. Global politics, including the implications of the UK's departure from the European Union, pose serious threats to animal welfare gains made in recent decades. I make reference to animal welfare standards in countries with whom the UK may strike trade deals in the coming years; deals which would threaten to undermine UK animal welfare standards if imports were not legally required to at least meet the same standards. Global markets mean that the animal welfare problems I discuss must be addressed by nations across the world, to help avoid individual countries raising their domestic standards but importing cheaper lower-standard products, thereby exporting the problems they had set out to address. We need a reimagined global food system, supported by engaged citizens rather than passive consumers, in which food is properly priced and valued, and the poorest are supported. Dietary shifts are occurring across the world, with much debate about healthy and sustainable consumption of meat and dairy products. Interest in vegetarianism and veganism is at an all-time high in several countries. Use of technology, such as meat produced from cell culture rather than large numbers of farmed animals, is set to play an increasing role. I fully expect that my topics and perspectives will assume quite different relevance in the coming years, given the intensity of public focus on how we should relate to our natural environment and our fellow sentient animals.

Animal welfare standards in the UK are among the highest in the world, with the UK being one of the six highest-ranking countries on the global Animal Protection Index. But despite this, as we shall see, important problems persist and we must all keep progressing if we are to meet the conditions of a good life and a humane death for the animals who provide us with so much.

One of the ways we can reflect animal sentience is through our thoughtful use of language. In this book I have aimed to not refer to sentient animals as 'it', but rather to use 'he' or 'she' where the animal's sex is known and to use 'they' where the sex is not known, including if referring to a single animal. I have often found that cattle veterinarians and dairy farmers do this naturally; for example, saying of a cow who can't stand, 'She can't get up,' rather than, 'It can't get up'. We might say of an inanimate object, like a cushion, 'It's on the sofa', but it would feel wrong to say the same of, say, a grandparent. In this way, our language conveys our belief in an individual's capacity to experience feelings: that is, their sentience. It is not my intention to dictate how people should speak and write about animals and I would be inconsistent in my own daily application of these principles, but I hope it may offer pause for thought.

On Formby Beach, my footprints turn to reflective pools beneath the incoming tide, reminding me that we can tread lightly for animals and wash away the worst. My veterinary training and career have given me insights and information on how we treat animals, on animal welfare and animal ethics. I do not have all the answers by a long shot, but in this book I can share with you what I have seen and learned.

CHAPTER 2

Australian zebra finches

The 12-mile Sefton coastline is the largest dune complex in England and one of the most important areas for nature conservation in Europe. Passing from north to south, it takes in the Ribble Estuary, with its wheeling thousands of wintering waterfowl; the Ainsdale and Birkdale Sandhills; Formby, with its pinewoods, red squirrels and sandy beach; past the Alt Estuary and down to the sleepless Liverpool docks. To the east, sprawling mosslands nestle in the coast's hinterland. The landscape and its rare wildlife have featured prominently in the local culture, including in the name of the Squirrels Football Club and in the crest of Formby High School, which incorporates a pine tree and the rippling waves of the sea.

As a teenager I worked in a small pet shop in the heart of Formby where, each week, a steady flow of pet owners and wildlife lovers crammed into an Aladdin's cave of pet paraphernalia. The shop twitched and twittered with living creatures: rabbits, guinea pigs, hamsters and gerbils near the floor, with budgerigars, canaries and small finches in cages above.

Food for wild garden birds was in demand and at peak times people queued out of the shop waiting for a bag of seed or nuts. Feeding garden birds is now a multimillion pound industry in the United Kingdom (estimated at £210 million a year), but an aspect of the pet shop interested me. Here were bird lovers who presumably, like me, derived great pleasure from the dazzling colours, calls and characteristics of the birds that chose to visit their gardens: confident robins, a familiar blackbird, jaunty blue tits and others for whom we have such fondness. People delighted in seeing those birds dart from the hedge to deftly extract a seed from their feeder, or ascend to rooftops to deliver the songs that bring summer evenings to a perfect close. Yet for the pet shop birds, life was quite different. Here, life for the budgerigars, canaries and finches was a tick-list world of scrubbed surfaces, topped-up seed bowls and freshly filled water drinkers, a bland nod to the birds' vibrant wild potential. I wondered what would happen if, one Saturday morning, people arrived to find the cages not filled with so-called 'cage birds', but with robins, blackbirds and blue tits. I was sure there would be shock, maybe outrage and letters of complaint. Was confinement acceptable for budgies but not blue tits?

Part of the answer derives from cultural influence. We are so accustomed to seeing species such as budgies in cages (and most people have never seen them wild in their native Australia) that to see them confined is perfectly normal. Blue tits, however, are associated with their nimble antics in the back garden, so seeing them confined would seem, to some, quite wrong. But why? If people felt upset seeing native garden birds living as pets in small cages, what would be the basis for their concern?

They might be concerned that it is illegal, which, if the birds were wild-caught, would be correct. But if the practice were legal, it is likely that people would still be unhappy.

Perhaps they would have conservation concerns, worried that

removing birds from the wild would cause populations to dwindle. This is possible, and unsustainable trapping for the pet trade is a contributory source of endangerment for many species across the world.

But the reason I imagined most people would find the situation unpalatable is that they would view confinement of garden birds as unkind. They would feel that such birds should be free to live in space, as they choose, and that to have this taken away would cause them to have an unhappy life. The people, I guessed, would be concerned for the animals' welfare. If this was the case, would such concern be justified, and why would such logic not apply to budgies, canaries and exotic finches?

Such questions were all rather hypothetical and within the mind of a teenager focussed on whether he was going to be able to afford a drink with his friends. But later, as a veterinary student, I received a modest scholarship to undertake an exploratory research project looking into the question of whether birds have compromised welfare in pet shop cages.

Utilising the Five Freedoms introduced in Chapter 1, and animal welfare science, I was able, with the support of my academic supervisors, to explore how caged birds might be faring under typical pet shop conditions. I was never going to provide all the answers, but there was the potential to open a window on what life might be like behind the cage bars.

The species I chose to study was the Australian zebra finch, one of the most common and readily available finches kept in captivity. Zebra finches are small, the size of a blue tit, with the intricate detail typical of so many birds across the world. They are jumpy and lively, squeaking like dogs' toys or, as some prefer, a toy trumpet. When the time is right, the male quivers and melds his squeaks, building them ecstatically to a rapid, hiccupy song.

I contacted my former high school, who agreed to let me erect my battery of pet shop-style cages in a disused outbuilding. The building had lain untouched for years and a weathered door swung in to cobwebs and calm, away from the shrieks and dinner bells of the school corridors. Discarded school desks, with cold metal frames, spread across the floor and reared up to the ceiling.

I spent several days moleing through the stored clutter, rearranging and disposing, until I had cleared a space that would house my cages. I positioned a stepladder, upon which I could sit to make my observations, and dragged a large old desk into place for my pens, pads and some small lamps. A week later the Finchery, as it came to be known, was echoing with the triumphant fanfares of 70 squeaking zebra finches.

For the first two weeks I spent each day watching the finches without formally recording any observations. The idea was that they should come to recognize my studious lank perched upon the stepladder and learn that I was not a threat. If I was to gain an insight into the birds' lives within the cages, I would have to be satisfied that they were relaxed in my presence and behaving in a way that I was not unduly influencing. Zebra finches are not naturally tame birds and I knew from working in the pet shop that when a cage was approached they would stop whatever they were doing and alight to the safety of their perches. Here they would remain alert and watchful, having ceased all previous activities, until they were confident that the source of their disturbance had passed. Then their apparent anxiety would thaw and their surprisingly rich social lives would resume, until, perhaps only minutes later, the next customer loomed large from the shop floor.

The process I was employing in the Finchery is called 'habituation', whereby through gradual repeated exposure an animal comes to be accustomed to something they initially perceived as threatening. It is the same as the process used in the jungles of Africa, where families of mountain gorillas now tolerate the daily close presence of awestruck eco-tourists, having become accustomed to months of patient contact from local guides and researchers. Without habituating the birds to my presence, as they did to the gorillas, I would not gain a reliable insight into their lives. Initially when I approached, they would emit alarm calls and flee to their perches as in the pet shop, but as the days wore on their responses reduced until eventually they continued to feed on the ground (where they are at their most vulnerable), court and interact freely in my company. During this habituation period, I was also able to begin writing shorthand codes to describe the various behaviours unfolding before me, which I would use to record their activities in the weeks ahead.

The birds' cages were of the type found in most pet shops to house a small number of birds: a rectangular box with two perches, a seed tub and tall water drinker clipped to the bars. I tended to the birds diligently, ensuring they were kept at the right temperature, well fed and their homes kept clean, but despite these provisions the question remained of whether the birds were experiencing a good quality of life within their cage confines. Applying the Five Freedoms, potential welfare problems were identified as follows:

- **Freedom from hunger and thirst**: The finches had a plentiful supply of nutritious food and fresh water so should not have been hungry or thirsty. No obvious problem was identified.

- **Freedom from discomfort**: The temperature in the Finchery was monitored and became neither too hot nor too cold. The smooth, uniform-diameter perches sold with many cages are a risk factor for poor foot health, and so I monitored for signs of problems.

- **Freedom from pain, injury or disease**: Aside from an initial outbreak of stress-related disease, the birds appeared to be in good health, showing no ongoing signs of pain, injury or disease. No obvious problem was identified.

- **Freedom to express normal behaviour**: It would be hard to describe the finches' behaviour within the cages as normal. In the wild, zebra finches may fly many miles across the grassland habitats of their extensive home range. They move in flocks, forming large communal roosts, while also utilizing separate social trees or bushes to rest, sing and preen themselves and each other. They have regular bathing sites and specific trees for post-bathing preening. It was difficult to recognize the 'highly social and mobile lives' of the zebra finch, as described by the late Australian ornithologist Dr Richard Zann, in the Finchery, not least since they would usually form a tight lifelong pair bond with a mate. My finches, however, were not wild, having been born in captivity. Did this change their needs relating to normal behaviour? Questions like this warranted further consideration and investigation.

- **Freedom from fear and distress**: The potential for repeated fearful experiences in pet shops, as customers peer into cages, has been described, but beyond the period of habituation in my experimental set-up, the finches did not show continued signs of fear or distress. Fear is typically shown by taking flight suddenly; flying in a panicked, uncontrolled manner; or freezing to a spot, poised with breathing movements that are visibly accelerated. No such signs were routinely visible in my finches, so no obvious problem was identified.

Given this analysis, I set out to explore whether zebra finches, despite apparently being provided with the majority of things they need, might be experiencing poor welfare on account of their inability to express normal behaviour, whatever this might be or mean.

Over a period of five weeks I became established as a constant feature within the finches' truncated wilderness, my hunched body upon the boughs of my stepladder before them and the occasional studious rustle from my leaves of notes. I arrived at the Finchery by bicycle at 9am each morning and commanded dawn with the flick of a switch. A volley of calls and songs erupted from the cages as a tungsten sunrise stirred the birds from their nightly huddles, then, after feeding and watering, I sat and watched their daily routines play out before me.

After a short while it was clear that several birds had found a partner with whom, as occurs in the wild, they spent the majority of their day. Pairs clump together (meaning they perch in close contact with one another), interspersing this contact with bouts of tender allopreening, in which one of the pair gently nibbles and preens the feathers around the head and neck of the other. They separate rarely and move around the cage as a closely bonded couple. These scenes of touching devotion, however, had some sinister undertones. Those birds who were not enjoying the companionship and apparent affection of a closely bonded partner became untouchables: finch society outcasts who had no place within the social circles of the bonded pairs. With little place to go, an untouchable would attempt to land on a perch, along from a happy couple, only to be displaced aggressively by one of the bonded pair who would fly at them and peck them viciously if they did not immediately flee. My observations revealed that, with nowhere to escape, these unbonded birds were, in some cases, being attacked for up to 24 per cent of their waking time, especially during the early part of the day, and the effect of this was reflected in their behaviour. The outcasts never relaxed, flicking their wings nervously and moving about persistently in an agitated manner. When they did finally find refuge, it was on the cage floor where they would spend disproportionately high amounts of time: a place where, as we have noted, perching birds feel naturally most vulnerable.

In the wild, such aggressive behaviour is, of course, perfectly normal and unbonded birds would emigrate to a different part of the widely spread colony, perhaps even to a new colony, until they became paired themselves. But the grip of confinement permitted no such escape. These birds had no place to go and one suffered feather loss from pecking by other birds to such an extent that I had to remove the victim on humane grounds. It may seem unkind to have subjected these small birds to such hardship, but my purpose, remember, was to replicate and understand the implications of keeping these finches in a way that is common in pet shops around the world.

My inquisitive vigil ceases at 5:30pm each evening, at which time I am able to abandon my own captivity. I leave the Finchery and, after a quick visit home for a meal, cycle through the leafy roads of Formby until my route reaches a point where the houses begin to peter out and I enter a lane running alongside some allotments. It is June and the summer evening air caresses my face as I pedal. The lane is bordered by hedgerows, upon which greenfinches and goldfinches momentarily alight before resuming their bounding flight paths across nearby gardens, then high up into the gods of towering poplars.

A narrow earthy footpath trails ahead in a beeline to the coast, as do so many in this area, bordered by a dyke and three large ploughed fields to the right and a narrow belt of planted pines to the left. Through these can be seen glimpses of the Ministry of Defence-owned Altcar Rifle Range.

I lock my bicycle to a fence and proceed down the track on foot. It is 9pm and the day is drawing to a close. The silence amplifies until the evening air begins to cool on my cheeks while the sun lowers further, and a cotton-wool acoustic begins to wrap around, leaving only the padding of my feet on soft earth and the muffled knocking of binoculars against my chest.

After around 200 metres, the dark line of pine trees comes to an end and the path bulbs slightly. Damp mud reflects the last of the day's light. I lean towards the spindly rushes, primed, after many summers visiting this location, to pluck treasure from this fantasy landscape. A thin high-pitched trilling begins to emanate from the undergrowth. The sound is continuous, like a pinhead delicately pulled across a long, ribbed, metallic radiator, end to end without pause, gathering in volume, then decreasing. Its source is perhaps just 5 metres away, but I can see nothing. I will the fading light into my binoculars and focus them on the densely clumped vegetation, examining stem by stem, but the originator of the sound remains concealed. All the while the trilling ripples through me. As the vast trillions of stars are most appreciable in one's peripheral vision, so the song of the grasshopper warbler might be imagined to inhabit one's 'peripheral hearing'. The sound is all about me, but ungraspable. I know the bird in the rushes is olive-brown, small and skulking, wary and reclusive. Slightly smaller than a dunnock, a bird of similarly unassuming characteristics, he has arrived to this careless tatter of tussocks from West Africa and most frequently produces his strange monotonous trill at dusk and dawn. I know the bird has climbed partway up a stem and is moving his head slowly from side to side as he sings; this behaviour explains the variation in intensity. I stop searching and just enjoy the sound. I am fond of my annual connection with the grasshopper warbler at this location, a bird I have barely ever seen but which adds to my familiarity and sense of belonging here. Grasshopper warblers travel the globe and are invisibly inconspicuous. They have been added to the UK red list of birds of highest conservation concern, due to significant population decline. For these few moments of strained, appreciative concentration, my human thoughts and concerns are elsewhere, while this bird's audible presence streams upon my reflective solitude once again at this time, in this very clump of grass, in this very ditch.

I press on a further 100 metres down the track, crossing the boundary into Cabin Hill National Nature Reserve. The rifle range now opens up fully on my left, with its strange vacant buildings and shelters used for training exercises, while to my right stretches the calm open water of Cabin Hill Lake. Standing on the path next to the lake, I am now at the centre of a whirling hirundine vortex. In the twilight I cannot make out individual insects above the lake, but their presence, dancing above the water, has attracted mesmeric hordes of late-flying swallows and martins. I try to watch an individual but am hopelessly distracted by others, my gaze switching from one, to one, to one. A swift, cutting through the base of the cyclone, screams past my ear, coming at me like the thundering arm of a human centrifuge. I am consumed by the dazzling mastery of flight, finding myself unable to think beyond circles and spheres. I am shackled at the centre of a wheeling avian gyroscope, lifted from the path and floating above the lake through the dusky sky, amid the crackles and raspberries of the blown-leaf house martins, and the accelerating screams of the sickle-blade swifts. I sit down on the soft vegetation just off the path, looking across the lake, and think about my zebra finches.

I had set out to ask questions about whether their welfare, or quality of life, was compromised through their inability to express normal behaviour in small cages. Why is it acceptable to cage a budgie but not a blue tit, I had wondered.

But are the two really that similar? Perhaps my question does not compare like with like. Perhaps there are important differences between canaries, budgies and zebra finches, compared with native species such as robins and blackbirds.

Among these differences, and perhaps the most likely to be proffered, is that canaries and budgerigars are domesticated, bred for generations in captivity by humans. According to this suggestion, robins and the like are wild untamed spirits, stripped of all potential when confined, whereas canaries and domesticated others, through selective breeding, are now adapted to their life behind bars.

A second idea is that thwarting natural behaviour does not, in itself, lead to suffering, in the way that physical disease or injury might.

Thirdly, there is the notion that wild animals may suffer if brought in to captivity as they might miss their former lifestyle, whereas animals born in captivity cannot suffer from behavioural restriction as they have never known anything different. Through animal welfare science, we now know that each of these suggestions is likely to be poorly founded.

Through studies of animal motivation it is known that animals, including those who have been domesticated over many generations, can have strong desires to perform certain key elements of their natural behaviour, even in captivity.

In their natural habitats, all animal species face many natural pressures and challenges, such as the need to find food, to avoid predators and to stay fit and healthy. Inevitably, those animals who are best suited to the habitat they are living in will survive, and will pass their successful traits, via their genes, to their offspring. This is the process known as survival of the fittest, which, over evolutionary time, leads to species becoming highly adapted to the natural environments that they live in.

There are several kinds of traits that result in an animal being suited to the habitat they are living in. An animal's anatomy might be particularly beneficial: for example, having a long beak that can extract nectar from the centre of long flowers. An animal's physiology also needs to be well suited to the environment: for example, the cardiorespiratory system of a seal allows them to make deep dives to hunt fish. Additionally, an animal's behaviour is important in determining that animal's suitability for their environment. For example, the sow who makes a safe, warm nest for her piglets is less likely to have her piglets found and killed by a predator. The genes for nest building will therefore be passed on to her offspring, until eventually nest-building behaviour will become the norm throughout the species (as, indeed, it has). This means that, like anatomy and physiology, behaviour is one of several traits that influence an animal's biological fitness and differential survival in their natural environment.

Behaviour, like other important traits, has a genetic basis – a heritable component – that can be passed from generation to generation, and this allows behaviour to evolve and influence survival. Of course, some behaviour is learned during the course of an animal's life, and lifetime experience has an important role to play in shaping behaviour. But some behaviour in all animals has a genetic component. When we see animals in the wild, be they squirrels, shrews or grasshopper warblers, they have all, over millions of years, become well adapted to life in the environments we find them, through such things as their anatomy, their physiology and their behaviour.

So how does this relate to our questions about zebra finch behaviour and wellbeing? The crucial thing to remember here is that domestic animals have rarely had their natural behaviour bred out of them. Domestication, occurring over thousands of years at most, is a mere blink on the evolutionary scale. While humans may have chosen to breed from animals who looked a particular way, so were aesthetically pleasing, or from those who grew particularly well so that they would yield more meat, such tweaking and tinkering of the animals' genetic make-up has rarely affected their natural behaviour. Even when animals have been selectively bred for certain behavioural traits, such as docility (to facilitate handling) or aggression (to guard livestock or property), the rest of their behavioural repertoire has remained largely unaltered. This means that, despite domestication, most animals are driven to behave in the way that their wild ancestors did millions of years ago. As Professor Per Jensen of Linköping University in Sweden writes:

> Although there are behavioural differences between wild and domestic animals, it is clear that these are not as large as we sometimes tend to believe. It is also frequently suggested that domestic animals are less responsive to their environment than are wild animals, and even that they are 'more stupid'. However, detailed studies of the behaviour of domestic animals in natural conditions reveal that their behaviour is very similar to that of their ancestors [...] We need to remember that the behaviour of domestic animals is controlled by genetic mechanisms shaped over thousands and thousands of generations of evolution in the wild, and only slightly altered during domestication. The evolutionary history and adaptations of their ancestors and the natural behaviour of the present-day animals are therefore important pieces of information if we want to understand the animals we keep for our benefit.

Or as Professor Marian Dawkins of the University of Oxford puts it:

> Domestic animals are not man-made for confinement. They bring with them an evolutionary legacy from the past.

Three fascinating examples illustrate this principle. The first is the example of pigs studied by animal welfare researchers Professor David Wood-

Gush and Dr Alex Stolba in Edinburgh, in the early 1980s. At this time, behaviourally restrictive farming systems had become widespread, and Stolba and Wood-Gush were interested in whether housing for pigs could be designed that would achieve acceptable productivity while allowing the pigs to behave naturally and removing the need for extreme confinement. To do this, the scientists first needed to find out which types of behaviour might be considered natural for domestic pigs, so they released pigs into a large enclosed area of wooded countryside near Edinburgh (which came to be known as the Edinburgh Pig Park) and recorded hundreds of hours of observations of the pigs' behaviour. Professor David Fraser reports on the researchers' findings:

> The pigs, despite being domesticated through hundreds of generations of artificial selection, proved to retain virtually all the behavioural repertoire of their wild ancestor, the European wild boar. The pigs lived in small groups of several sows and their offspring. They spent hours per day rooting in the soil [...] They used dunging areas well removed from their resting areas. And when a sow was about to give birth, she would move away from the social group and build an elaborate nest in a secluded, partly hidden area where she would remain with the new litter for several days before rejoining the social group.

The second example comes from rats. Rats used for scientific research often live in shoebox cages (the name gives a clue to their dimensions) and, like domestic pigs, have also been bred for hundreds of generations in captivity. Dr Manuel Berdoy, a researcher at the University of

Oxford, wanted to know to what extent wild-type behaviour remained, unexpressed, in the domestic laboratory rat. To find out, he released a group of them into a large outdoor enclosure. Here they had to 'compete, like their wild cousins, for food, shelter and mates'. The rats' behaviour was recorded and formed a half-hour film, *The Laboratory Rat: A Natural History*. The 50 rats that were released were born and raised in a laboratory and had been domesticated for generations, but, just like the pigs, a complex and structured society soon emerged, with the rats behaving just like their wild ancestors. They explored, took shelter, dug in the earth and hopped – all behaviours that had been impossible in their shoebox cages. Of the experiment's relevance to animal welfare, Berdoy wrote:

> When keeping animals in captivity, it is important to know what they have evolved to do. Progress in animal welfare is, to a large extent, driven by a combination of awareness, willingness and facts. This film aims to be relevant to all three by reviewing the range of behaviours and needs which, despite generations of domestication, remain innate and ready to be expressed when given the opportunity.

The third example comes from chickens. There has been a rise in popularity of people keeping hens in their back garden, and many are electing to give a home to commercial laying hens who have spent their life in a cage. The birds arrive scruffy and poorly feathered, having never seen life beyond the farm shed, and they hesitantly explore their new surroundings. But within days, the same finding as is seen with the domestic pigs and rats is once again played out. The hens quickly form a wild-type social hierarchy and roam about their new space performing the same behaviour as their ancestral species, the red jungle fowl, scratching in the earth, dust bathing and perching at night. Even if they have never had access to a perch or a substrate to dust bathe in before, their innate motivation to utilize such resources, evolved over millennia, rapidly finds expression. As they roll from side to side in a dusty depression, flicking the earth upon themselves with their feet, and fluffing and flapping their wings to distribute the beneficial particles through their plumage, it is difficult not to feel sadness that millions of laying hens across the world will never have such opportunity in their restrictive wire mesh cages.

But is such regret warranted? These examples tell us that domesticated animals who have only ever experienced life in captivity will readily behave like their wild ancestors when given the opportunity to do so, and they imply that caged zebra finches would also behave like their wild Australian counterparts if they were released into large, naturalistic enclosures. But does this mean that confined animals want to behave in a different way when their space and opportunity is restricted, leading to a poor quality of life or suffering when they cannot? And does it mean that the only way to adequately provide for an animal's wellbeing is to allow them to perform their full range of species-specific behaviour?

Thanks to animal welfare science, we are beginning to be able to answer questions like these. To give a summary answer, it would seem that some behaviours are more important to animals than others (which behaviours depends on the species) and if the animal cannot perform these particular behaviours suffering can result. Conversely, being given choices and opportunities to perform normal behaviours in their living environments can contribute to a good quality of life.

The scientific approach leading to such an answer was developed by Professor Marian Dawkins. In the early 1980s, Dawkins developed experiments that 'asked' animals how much they want to perform certain behaviours when they are captive and proposed consumer demand theory as a way of understanding the animals' answers. Dawkins' approach can be explained as follows.

If a single species of animal is watched for many painstaking hours, human observers can formulate a list of all the behaviours that animal performs. When observing my zebra finches, for example, I recorded behaviours such as hopping, pecking, flying, eating, preening, aggressive jabbing and so on. When a species has been observed for long enough, there comes a point when no further behaviours can be added. That is to say, there is a finite number of behaviours that any individual species can and does perform. This is called the behavioural repertoire for that species and the list of recorded behaviours is known as the ethogram.

Dawkins wanted to examine whether animals were motivated to perform some behaviours in their repertoire more than others, and whether this could inform conclusions about their wellbeing. Based on her early experiments with hens, whom she trained to choose between different resources (such as litter in which to dust bathe versus food), she proposed that an animal's desire to do or have certain things could be interpreted using theory from economics.

This may sound off-putting, but it is quite simple. Economic theory says that when times get tough, people will continue to buy certain things but will stop buying others. As income drops (perhaps because someone in the family has lost their job) or prices rise, families may continue to buy bread (a so-called commodity) but may forego an expensive holiday (a so-called luxury). Commodities are said to demonstrate inelastic demand, whereas luxuries show elastic demand. This is the basis of consumer demand theory.

By training animals to perform tasks to access resources (for example pressing a lever or pushing through a weighted door to get to something they want on the other side), experiments can be designed that allow the same theory to be applied. By manipulating how much effort must be put in to the task (for example by increasing the number of presses they must do, or increasing the weight they must push through), the 'price' of accessing the resource can be raised. Reducing 'income' can be achieved by reducing the amount of time an animal is given to perform a task. When experiments of this nature are conducted, it is found that animals will keep lever-pressing or will push through doors of ever-increasing weight to access some resources, whereas for other resources they will quickly give up. This gives us information about how much the animals want to get to the resource. Experiments like this reveal that animals are highly motivated to gain access to some environments (they show inelastic demand), whereas other environments are not so important to them (showing elastic demand). A certain environment may be important to the animal because it contains a resource that they need or want very much (such as food when they are hungry), or because it allows them to perform a certain behaviour which requires a certain environmental feature (such as perching, which requires a perch).

An experiment with American mink, published in the leading journal *Nature*, gives an example of this approach.

Wild mink live in burrows near to water, and males may occupy around 2,500 acres of wetland habitat. They mark their territory by scent-marking in prominent locations and are semi-aquatic, being able to dive to a depth of 5 metres using their partially webbed feet. In contrast, mink farmed for their fur are raised in small wire mesh cages, with limited opportunity to perform any of their normal behaviour. Professor Georgia Mason and her colleagues at the University of Guelph sought to determine whether farmed mink were frustrated in their barren wire cages – specifically, whether there were certain natural behaviours they had a strong desire to perform that the cage did not permit. They housed mink in conventional farm cages and attached seven similarly sized compartments containing different resources:

> A water pool measuring about 1.5 x 0.5 m and filled with 0.2 m water; a raised platform, reached by a 2 m vertical wire tunnel; novel objects such as traffic cones and packaging, which were changed daily; an alternative nest site (a box of hay); toys for manipulation and chewing (tennis balls, for example); and a plastic tunnel. The seventh compartment was left empty to control for the importance of simply making extra space available.

The mink were able to access the various compartments by passing through weighted doors, and the weight was systematically increased over six weeks. By automatically recording the animals' behaviour day and night, the researchers found that the mink were highly motivated to access the water pool and rated it as the most valuable resource. They pushed through greater and greater weights to access it (showing inelastic demand) and they pushed through a higher weight to reach the pool than for any other resource.

This showed that fur-farmed mink have a strong desire to be able to swim. But what of the second question: do animals who show such strong desires suffer in captivity if they are unable to perform these highly motivated behaviours? To answer this, motivation experiments such as these need to be coupled with measures of animal stress when the animals are prevented from performing the highly motivated behaviour. In the case of the mink, once the researchers had discovered that the animals had a strong desire to access water, they then blocked access to the water pool and measured the stress hormone, cortisol, in the mink's urine. It rose as high as it does when they are temporarily prevented from accessing food. The cortisol rise was much less marked when they were prevented from accessing the other resources that they had worked less hard to reach in the first experiment. In this example, just one stress indicator, cortisol, was measured, but in other experiments other indicators have also been measured to provide extra validity. Based on their findings, Mason's team drew the following conclusions:

Our results indicate that fur-farmed mink are still motivated to perform the same activities as their wild counterparts, despite being bred in captivity for 70 generations, being raised from birth in farm conditions, and being provided with food [constantly]. The high level of stress experienced by mink denied access to the pool, rated as the most valuable resource, is evidenced by an increase in cortisol production indistinguishable from that caused by food deprivation. These results suggest that caging mink on fur farms does cause the animals frustration, mainly because they are prevented from swimming.

Mason highlighted the argument made by the fur farming industry that mink have adapted to life in captivity, as judged by their good health and breeding success, but she concluded, as has been noted earlier in this chapter, that good physical health is not enough. It is necessary, but not sufficient. Animals, like the mink, as well as being healthy, also need to be able to perform certain aspects of their natural behaviour. If they cannot, the evidence suggests they will suffer.

The last of the house martins spiralled up into the now dark sky, their airspace quickly filled by the scatty flight of pipistrelle bats. The information relevant to my finches passed through my mind: animals do not need to perform all of the behaviours in their behavioural repertoire, but there are some behaviours that if they cannot perform can lead to frustration and a poor quality of life. I contemplated which of my zebra finches' behaviours might fall in to this category but was aware that the focus of such experiments has yet to fall on this species; animal welfare science is less than 60 years old and the welfare of farmed animals and laboratory rodents has thus far taken priority.

Some of these highly motivated behaviours have been referred to as behavioural needs, because actually doing the behaviour is more important to the animal than the end result of having done it. Sows, for example, if given a pre-formed nest very similar in composition to one they would construct for themselves, still perform nest-building behaviour shortly before farrowing. The term 'behavioural need' is considered to apply to behaviours that are highly motivated as a result of internal mechanisms, such as those controlled by hormones (as in the case of nest building in sows). Some behaviour is mainly motivated by external factors, such as aggression or predator avoidance. An animal will not usually behave aggressively, or flee, unless they are confronted by an aggressor or a predator. Therefore, such an animal in captivity will not suffer if they cannot perform these behaviours. But if the animal has a build-up of motivation due to internal influences, they will become frustrated and may suffer if their environment provides no opportunity for those behaviours to be performed.

As I made my way back along the path I considered other criteria proposed by Marian Dawkins as being potentially useful in categorising certain behaviours as behavioural needs, and wondered if I had encountered them in my birds. Dawkins noted that if animals are very highly motivated to behave in certain ways, they may behave abnormally if their captive environment prevents them from performing those behaviours. The presence, then, of these abnormal behaviours could indicate that highly motivated behaviour has been thwarted, which may be linked to suffering.

The first abnormal behaviour is called vacuum behaviour. Vacuum behaviour is behaviour that animals perform even when the usual stimuli for that behaviour are not present: for example, animals may behave as though building a nest, even when no nesting material is present.

The second possible sign of a frustrated behavioural need is rebound behaviour. This is behaviour that occurs at a higher than normal level when it is finally permitted. In some cases it appears that, during the period of deprivation, the internal motivation to behave in a certain way becomes stronger and stronger, in the same way that an animal's motivation to drink becomes stronger when they cannot access water. When the opportunity finally presents itself, as in the case of drinking water when very thirsty, the animal performs the behaviour at a higher than usual level.

Thirdly, stereotypic behaviours (or stereotypies) are fixed behavioural sequences performed repetitively, which serve no obvious function. Examples familiar to many come from animals in zoos and circuses, including polar bears pacing repetitively in their concrete enclosures and captive elephants who sway their head and trunk from side to side for hours on end. When the performance of highly motivated behaviour is prevented, these deranged behavioural sequences may be the consequence.

I had noticed some unusual behaviours in some of my birds, but I was keen to investigate whether they could be categorized as any of these abnormal behaviours in particular. This, I thought, might shed some further light on whether my zebra finches were unhappy in their cages and I pursued this over the coming weeks.

My 70 birds came to the end of their time in the high school Finchery at the end of my five-week study and I was able to rehome all of them to spacious, enriched aviaries. As the cages stood silent and empty, I undertook my nightly passage to Formby Beach to reflect upon what I had seen and learnt.

I pass through the dunes once more on to the vast, sandy stage beyond. High tide is just receding and the sea is close and still. An absence of people in any direction creates a perfect unbroken horizon as it awaits the dipping sun. As usual, I feel privy to a private viewing, but a small audience take their vantage point from the water: the heads of three grey seals visible, then disappearing.

I cycle south along the firm sand, to a beach entrance point at Lifeboat Road. Black and white photographs show bearded men and great horses hauling a timber boat into foaming waves. Now, just a square frame of red bricks penetrating through the sand is all that remains of Britain's first lifeboat station, established here in 1776. On an evening like this it is hard to conceive of the need for it, but I have also experienced the fury of violent storms.

Next to the worn foundations of the lifeboat station are the remains of a brick chimney-like column, lying at a 45-degree angle towards the open sky. I place my bike on the soft sand and sit in the mouth of the column, facing the sea.

The beach is perfectly silent. In the distance I can see the brilliant white of gannets patrolling above the waves in search of fish. Closer in, Sandwich and common terns carry their ribbon tails through the sea air with elegant thrusting wings; the creaking-gate 'kear-iks' from the Sandwich terns are the only sound to carry. Dotted about the sky, small, wheeling flocks of migrating wading birds – sanderling, bar-tailed godwits, dunlin and oystercatchers – touch soft brush strokes across the sunset's blushing cheeks.

I think of my zebra finches. In my pet shop-style cages I had found that these gregarious birds had formed pair bonds as they would in the wild. This, however, led to high levels of aggression towards unbonded birds who could not escape the attacks due to space restrictions imposed by the cages. Some of these victims were bullied and severely feather-pecked. Despite forming strong pair bonds, finches are sold indiscriminately, often according to the aesthetic preferences of consumers, so bonds are likely to be frequently broken. Is this distressing for them? Further research would be required to investigate this, but it was notable that when one of my bonded birds escaped from his cage into the Finchery one day, each of the pair vocalized constantly to one another, while the behaviour of both birds was agitated until they were reunited. When male guinea pigs are separated from their colony, their stress response is significantly lower when they are accompanied by their bonded female, compared to when they are removed on their own or with females to whom they are not bonded. The question of whether zebra finches may be distressed by enforced separation would be open to similar scientific examination.

I also found that over 10 per cent of my birds by the end of the five-week study had developed abnormal behaviours, of the kinds associated with thwarted behavioural needs. Some had developed vacuum nesting behaviour. In the 30 minutes preceding lights off at the end of the day, they would sit on the cage floor performing nest-building actions in the absence of nesting material. This finding makes it quite plausible that zebra finches have a behavioural need to build nests, a conclusion which is supported by knowledge of their natural history; zebra finches are one of ten Australian species belonging to the Estrildidae family that build a nest specifically for roosting purposes.

Others developed stereotypic behaviour. Some performed spot picking – repeatedly touching a particular spot on the side of the cage – while others developed repetitive route tracing – repeatedly following a precise and unvarying route within their cage, similar to pacing wolves. Such stereotypic behaviours have previously been described by researchers studying canaries (another species of finch) in the 1960s, and hopping and flying from a perch in a circle back to the same perch was postulated as being stereotypic by a team of researchers studying zebra finches at the UK's Royal Veterinary College in the mid-1990s.

Finally, when my finches were offered water baths they appeared to relish the opportunity to bathe. The highest number of birds (96 per cent of them) bathed on the first day that baths were introduced and the time it took them to first jump in was also lowest on the day that baths were first introduced, indicating a strong desire to access bathing water when it was made available. It is possible that such behaviour could be classed as rebound behaviour, revealing a build-up of internal motivation to splash water through their unwashed feathers.

My foray into the lives of caged zebra finches was a mere pilot study, but what I saw over the preceding weeks raised my concerns that, despite being 'well looked after', the wellbeing of zebra finches may not be adequately catered for in the small unstimulating cages that frequently become their homes. This endearing and beautiful bird is kept both for pleasure and as the avian model of choice in an array of scientific disciplines. Despite this, the eminent authors of *The UFAW Handbook on the Care and Management of Laboratory and Other Research Animals* note that 'it is surprising that very little work has been conducted on their welfare'.

Having shared many moments with these birds, and knowing of the many other bird species that are similarly caged around the world, I can only hope this is something that will be rectified through continuing public support for charities like the Universities Federation for Animal Welfare (UFAW) who funded my study and publically funded research councils.

Investigations such as mine have the potential to yield objective insights into the quality of lives of animals, but their conclusions do not tell us whether the way we choose to keep and treat animals is right or wrong. For this, we must interpret our findings in the context of our value systems and question how they fit within our ethical frameworks. If scientifically rigorous observation gives evidence for poor wellbeing in caged zebra finches, is this harm justified by the hedonistic gains they bring to bird keepers?

As the sun finally disappears beyond the horizon and the last of the terns disperse into the darkening skies, I recall the words of Robert MacFarlane, commenting on the beauty of wild bearded tits and providing insight into his own ethical leaning:

> The charm of these birds has cost them though [...] I find it difficult to see why anyone would want to cage one of these exquisite, spirited birds. They belong out here in this landscape of freedom, movement and flight.

CHAPTER 3

Herons and hens

My cycle rides and evening meanders around Formby typically gravitate towards the coast because I am drawn to the beach like the tide itself. But sometimes I head inland, across the mosslands. The landscape is flat and wild, but more visibly managed than the coast, with its plough-furrowed fields and man-made drainage channels.

From home, I pass through the built environment, then cross the Formby Bypass, a busy artery flowing along the town's easterly border. Immediately I enter the open landscape of telegraph wires and patchwork fields, where regimented rows of crops form fibrin-like lattices, sealing me in to the hushed open space beyond the haemorrhaging roar of traffic. After a short stretch crossing Formby Moss along a track, I join the Cheshire Lines Path, a disused railway line forming part of the Trans Pennine Trail. From here onwards I am able to pedal through quiet, open countryside.

The buildings in which we rear some animals for their meat and eggs are commonly long, low and nondescript, such as those on the poultry farm I am bound for. Sometimes I see these buildings from a train, but

I doubt whether those around me know what is inside them.

As our societies become more urbanized, we become further removed from the reality of where and how our food is produced. Many shoppers are unlikely to associate a cut of cellophane-wrapped meat in a plastic tray with the animal from which it came; indeed, some actively reject any meat products which could still be identified as a dead animal. Reported surveys have suggested that nearly a quarter of UK adults don't know that bacon comes from pigs and a quarter of 8–11 year old children think cheese comes from a plant.

Most of us live our lives physically distant from the agricultural environment. Farm animal buildings exist in the middle of nowhere; they are off our radar. But we, the food-purchasing public, are becoming more informed about the ethical issues raised alongside livestock. This is critical if, as civilized societies, we are to collectively determine an ethically acceptable farming future.

In the UK, laying hens were typically kept as relatively small, free-range flocks with movable huts until the 1950s, when the use of cages became popular, driven by the demand for cheap food in the post-war period. Hens kept for commercial egg production were then widely housed in small, barren, battery cages until 1999, when an EU-wide ban on such cages for laying hens was introduced, with a total phase-out by 2012. EU countries must now use the 'furnished' or 'enriched' cage, which additionally provides a perch, nest box and scratching area. Approximately half of the laying hens in Europe (equating to over 175 million birds) are currently housed in these cages, with 36 per cent of eggs from the UK's 39 million laying hens coming from birds kept in this way. The bare wire battery cage is still used to house around 4.5 billion of the approximately 7.5 billion laying hens globally, accounting for an estimated 70 per cent of laying hens in the US (over 200 million birds in cages), 66 per cent of laying hens in Canada (17 million birds in battery cages), half of laying hens in Australia (11 million birds in battery cages) and over 90 per cent of laying hens in China, the world's biggest egg producer (2.8 billion birds in cages). The widespread use of barren battery cages around the world risks hampering further animal welfare progress in the UK post-Brexit, if imports through trade deals with these countries are permitted to undermine current UK standards.

Stepping inside a shed of battery hens for the first time is an unforgettable experience. Prior to the EU ban on the unenriched system – but bearing in mind this still accounts for 60 per cent of global laying hen accommodation – I visited an intensive farm containing hundreds of thousands of laying hens housed in bare wire cages. I walked up a long drive towards the nearest of several long, low buildings. Swallows swooped around the farm buildings, chattering. Two German shepherd dogs came barking and bounding towards me, followed by a man wearing an old check shirt, worn-out trousers and wellingtons.

When we entered the closest building, there was an audible din coming from beyond a pair of closed doors. First I was taken to a quiet processing area where thousands of eggs spun upon rollers on conveyor belts for grading, sorting and packing. The farmer talked me through the various stages of the production process, pulling laminated charts from the wall to apprise me of performance data and targets. Then we walked back to the double doors and entered the shed.

The first thing to strike me was the noise. This building alone contained 55,000 hens, although battery sheds can contain over twice this number. To put this into perspective, Anfield, home to Liverpool Football Club with a reputation as one of the loudest stadia in the world, has a crowd capacity of 54,000.

As I looked into the metal cages next to me, I could pick out the voices of individual birds. Next was the sound of their movement, of their scaly feet and claws on the mesh cage floor, the tinny chinks of the cages vibrating against one another like instruments tuning discordantly before a symphony. But the expectant hush and harmonious perfection never followed. The din continued, as I walked deeper into the shed.

The farmer left me alone and I stood in the very heart of the clamouring, clattering, fever-pitch building. The cages around me were cramped, each containing five hens with a living ground space of just 550 square centimetres: an area well publicized as being less than a sheet of A4 paper. There were cages down at the level of my legs, continuing high up to the roof, requiring a ladder for inspection. Moving conveyors maintained a constant stream of food past the front of every cage and eggs rolled down perfectly engineered slopes for collection. Everywhere I looked I was being watched, examined; tens of thousands of beady eyes peering out at me from jerky heads. As I stood fixated, I thought of Ruth Harrison's *Animal Machines*: hens confined in battery cages, which the British Veterinary Association, responding to the government's subsequent inquiry, said it deplored.

I left the shed, thanked the farmer for his time and stepped back into the sunshine. After a short journey on my bicycle, I was back on the open mosslands. With a farmhouse just visible in the far distance, I pulled my

bike up on to a grassy embankment next to a brook, sat down next to it
and listened to the breeze blowing through the crops.

The life of a caged hen runs roughly as follows: chicks hatch in specialized
breeding units where eggs are automatically incubated in a tightly
controlled environment. The chicks are sexed and vaccinated against
serious diseases. Male chicks of laying hens have no commercial value since
they do not lay eggs and their slow growth makes them unsuitable for meat
production, so they are killed at one day old using either exposure to gas
or instantaneous mechanical destruction (maceration). Approximately
30 million chicks are killed like this in the UK each year. Before the females
are ten days old (the legal limit) many have their beak trimmed to reduce
feather and skin damage caused by feather pecking and cannibalism; in
the UK, this is performed using a high-intensity infrared beam. Elsewhere
in the world, it is still permissible to use a more painful hot blade.

Female chicks are purchased by poultry farmers when they are a day
old, reared to the age they begin laying eggs – around 18 weeks old – then
transported to another farm and placed in a cage where they will stay for
the rest of their life. Laying hens have been selectively bred to produce
eggs rapidly and efficiently, nearly an egg a day. This continues until they
are about 18 months old, when their egg production falls and they are
slaughtered. Because they have been bred for egg production, laying
hens are scrawny with little meat, which is used in soups, pastes and
pet foods.

Battery farming is a cheap and effective way of producing millions
of eggs every day. A poultry farmer was asked by a BBC reporter inside
a battery shed: 'When you look at this... are you OK with this now?'

The farmer cited the proposed benefits of battery cages, adding, 'People keep pet birds in cages, don't they?'

Laying hens have been among the most studied animals since animal welfare science began, and the findings have led to significant changes within the poultry industry. As for our analysis of caged-bird welfare in the previous chapter, the Five Freedoms can highlight welfare risks for caged hens.

1. Freedom from hunger and thirst

Hens in cages have constant access to nutritious food and plentiful water. Most of the time they should be neither hungry nor thirsty.

2. Freedom from discomfort

Thermal comfort: the hens are maintained at a comfortable temperature.

Physical comfort: the birds live on a wire mesh floor which can cause poor foot health. In barren battery cages they have nowhere comfortable to rest. With so little space they are unable to move about normally, for example to perform so-called comfort behaviours including wing stretching and flapping. Limited wing flapping is possible in the larger enriched cage and the hens have increased headroom in these cages.

3. Freedom from pain, injury or disease

Important infectious diseases of laying hens are well controlled by routine vaccination. Cages are cleaner than non-cage systems, as droppings fall through the floor and are removed. The air also tends to be less dusty, as no litter is present.

A significant health issue in all laying hens is that of osteoporosis (weak bones) and bone fractures. Fractures are painful and those affecting the keel bone (the breastbone) have been estimated to afflict approximately half of all laying hens in the UK (potentially affecting around 19.5 million birds), described as one of the most important welfare problems affecting commercial laying hens. Keel fractures occur in laying hens whether housed in cages or not.

Osteoporosis is seen in laying hens for two principal reasons. The first is their high productivity. To lay an egg a day places a huge demand on the hen's reserves of calcium. Calcium is needed to produce an egg shell, but also for strong, healthy bones. When more calcium is diverted to their eggs and insufficient calcium goes to their bones, the hen's bones become weak and brittle as a result.

The second reason is inactivity. To be healthy, bones need to have normal forces passing through them, which occurs during normal walking, hopping, wing flapping and other exercise. In the confines of a cage, normal movement is impossible and the bones weaken. Laying hens are therefore susceptible to fractures when they are handled during depopulation – when they are caught and removed from farm buildings at the end of their productive laying period.

Another important source of pain and injury for laying hens in cages and non-caged systems is injurious pecking. This is a collective term used to describe feather pecking, vent pecking and cannibalistic pecking, in which (as the names imply) hens peck at each other's feathers and vent (the anus), sometimes causing severe damage and death. Birds displaying this behaviour may be seen to start pecking repeatedly at an individual, who has nowhere to escape to when confined in a cage. This can continue until internal organs are reached and the bird dies. Feather pecking is not necessarily an aggressive behaviour; it is complex and unpredictable, suggested to be associated with stress and boredom. A single cause has not been found, but risk factors include rearing conditions, diet, lack of materials to forage in (which are nil in a battery cage), and the knowledge and management practices of stockpeople, who care for the birds.

A third source of pain for the majority of hens, previously mentioned, is beak trimming. Beak trimming involves cutting sensitive tissue that contains a high density of nerves. It is classed as a mutilation under British and European law, but is permitted to prevent injurious pecking.

4. Freedom to express normal behaviour

As was the case with my zebra finches, it would seem that one of the most obvious concerns regarding hens in cages is their extreme confinement and, in battery cages, the absence of any resources they would value, such as perches. The results of various experiments reveal that hens are highly motivated to roost on a perch at night, to perform nesting behaviour, to dust bathe, and to scratch and forage on the ground.

To 'ask' hens how much they wanted a nest site to lay their egg in, Professors Jonathan Cooper and Michael Appleby, then at the University of Edinburgh, provided their hens with littered, enclosed nest boxes. These were divided from a home pen containing food, water and a perch. To enter the nest box, the hens had to pass through a vertical gap which the experimenters varied in width from 22 centimetres to 9.5 centimetres. The mean body width of the hens was 11.7 centimetres. This meant that to pass through the narrowest gaps, the birds had to struggle and squeeze. At times when the birds were not going to lay an egg, they would casually enter and exit the nest box when the gaps were wide, but would stop doing this as the gaps became narrower (sometimes after a limited attempt to squeeze through). But in the two hours prior to laying an egg, all of the hens persevered in squeezing through. Cooper and Appleby concluded 'Hens were willing to pay a high cost to gain access to a nest box prior to [egg-laying], so pre-laying behaviour may be frustrated in hens without a well-defined, littered nest site.'

As is the case for most behavioural needs, this result should not come as a surprise when we consider the pre-laying behaviour of hens under natural conditions. Approximately 90 minutes before egg-laying, a hen seeks out a concealed location where she scrapes out a shallow hollow in the ground and builds a nest. This behaviour improves the reproductive success of the nest-building bird in the wild (for example, a clutch of eggs that is concealed is less likely to be predated or exposed to extreme climatic conditions), so the genes for nest-building behaviour are passed from generation to generation. As was noted in the previous chapter, such wild-type behaviour remains intact in the animals we keep and use today, despite generations of domestication.

A second, similar experiment looked at the possible frustration of hens prevented from accessing a perch to roost on at night. Free-living hens, like their wild ancestor the red jungle fowl, roost on branches in trees at night. Dr Anna Olsson and Professor Linda Keeling, working in Sweden, kept hens in littered pens with perches of varying heights and monitored their behaviour when the lights were turned off. At lights out, the birds began to ascend to the perches immediately and, within 10 minutes, more than 90 per cent of them were roosting close together on the top perch. The researchers then denied the hens access to the perches, either by covering the perches with a sloping board of plexiglass (so that they could see them, but would slide down if they attempted to perch on them) or by removing the previously available perches altogether. Under these conditions, the birds walked around their pen restlessly and took a long time to settle. Olsson and Keeling reported that the hens paced along the walls of the pen, repeatedly looking up at the walls, while others attempted to fly. Some pecked at their own feathers, which is also observed when access to food is prevented. The results, they wrote, 'imply that hens kept under conditions where perching is not possible may experience reduced welfare'.

Olsson and Keeling conducted a second series of experiments to see if hens would be willing to work to gain access to a perch. Initially, food was temporarily withheld from the birds and they were trained to push through weighted doors to access food on the other side. This revealed what the maximum resistance was that the birds would push through (they would push harder and harder as they became hungrier). Perches were then made available at night, and the birds, again, had to push through the weighted doors to reach them. If a perch was not of great importance to them they would have given up trying, but Olsson and Keeling found that they would push through a weight that was 75 per cent of the weight they would overcome to reach food when hungry. This was the first experiment to quantify how important perches are to hens for roosting.

Informed by findings such as these, a large EU-funded project on the welfare of laying hens – which was described as 'severely compromised' in conventional cages – reported that:

Our current knowledge indicates that the most important deficiency from the birds' perspective is the lack of provision of a discrete, enclosed nesting area. Nesting is a behavioural priority for laying hens. Moreover, perching, dust bathing and foraging are also very important parts of the normal behavioural repertoire that cannot be (fully) expressed in conventional cages.

5. Freedom from fear and distress

Physiological stress levels are higher in birds who are subjected to close confinement, and the frustration of several behavioural needs (as described above) is also likely to be distressing. Human handling during depopulation will lead to considerable fear and distress in both cage and non-cage systems.

Given the welfare problems associated with housing hens in cages, the practice has consistently received criticism. With widespread consensus about the harms caused to battery hens in particular, why has global society deemed it acceptable to farm them in this way?

There may be low awareness of mental wellbeing and behavioural needs in hens among the public and even some poultry farmers, who may think that as long as the hens are safe, warm and well fed, they must be fine. Another plausible explanation is that many people may have a low natural affinity and empathy for chickens, with some even viewing them as stupid. Such a view is entirely unwarranted and it can be seen from the experiments cited in this chapter that these are birds with preferences and an ability to readily learn new tasks.

Based on findings such as these and her own work on the chicken brain, Lesley Rogers, Emeritus Professor of Neuroscience and Animal Behaviour at the University of New England in Australia, wrote: 'With increased knowledge of the behaviour and cognitive abilities of the chicken has come the realization that the chicken is not an inferior species to be treated merely as a food source.' Put simply, chickens are thinking, feeling animals.

I looked along the line of the brook to see a grey heron lifting from the embankment, trailing marionette limbs as they strained towards the falling sun. The waterbird's slow wing beats mapped onto my spirit. Yet herons are birds of patient elegance, not weariness, and there is hope in the story of the battery hen.

Hens want to lay their eggs in a private space, to perch, dust bathe and forage, and to derive enjoyment from their surroundings.

Although laying hens are able to perform more of their natural behaviours in an enriched cage, the space afforded to them is still viewed as inadequate by many. Instead of a living space of 550 square centimetres in the conventional battery cage, the enriched cage provides more headroom and 750 square centimetres to each hen, 600 of which must be 'usable' (so that space must not include areas like nest boxes). An average of 600 square centimetres of usable ground space is still less than a sheet of A4 paper per bird. But how do the alternatives to enriched cages compare?

Since 2004, European Union law has required that all eggs must be labelled according to their system of production. These are: eggs from caged hens, barn eggs, free-range eggs and organic. Unfortunately, legislation does not prohibit the misleading use of pictures of rolling hills and green fields on caged and barn boxes – environments that neither a battery hen nor a barn hen would ever experience.

Barn eggs are produced by hens living in large houses, with each house often containing several thousand birds. The hens live on a floor covered with deep litter (such as wood shavings) with space to exercise and access to perches and nest boxes. The floor litter allows them to scratch, forage and dust bathe, though must be well managed to remain hygienic. The most common barn design, known as 'aviaries' in Europe, comprises multiple levels with feed, water, perches and nest boxes provided on each.

Free-range housing is similar to barn accommodation, but the barn contains multiple exit points – called 'pop holes' – along its sides. These allow the hens to go out in to a field where they can roam. Free-range is the only housing system that meets the requirements of the European Union regulation governing organic farming. Beak trimming is prohibited under organic systems and certain other organic requirements must be met; for example, the birds must have more floor and ranging space, their feed must be organic and the land that the hens are housed on must not have been treated with any synthetic fertilizers, herbicides or pesticides.

These non-cage systems also have their disadvantages. For example, to be one among thousands of hens in a free-range shed is quite unnatural in its own right, and the birds, who can be naturally aggressive (hence the term pecking order), may find it difficult to get from the centre of the shed to the pop holes at the edges. Twenty-five years ago, free-range flocks typically contained around 2,000–4,000 hens; today, 32,000 would be common, with many free-range flocks even larger than that.

Free-range birds are vulnerable to predation (such as by foxes and birds of prey), though this risk can be reduced by providing shelter and electric fencing. Caged hens tend to have a lower risk of infectious diseases and lower levels of internal parasites such as parasitic worms, as well as a lower risk of feather pecking and cannibalism. Feather pecking may be reduced because the hens are kept in small social groups, rather than having to maintain stable relationships with much larger numbers of surrounding birds in barns and free-range units. However, this practice is also linked to the birds' genetics and how they are managed by stockpeople. It has long been believed, based on available evidence, that mortality rates are higher for hens not housed in cages. However, a large-scale study published in the journal *Scientific Reports* in 2021 found that mortality in indoor cage-free housing decreases over time, until there are no differences between caged and non-caged systems. Using data from 16 countries, 6,040 commercial flocks and 176 million hens, the researchers demonstrated the benefits of farm managers gaining experience and knowledge of non-cage systems over time, coupled with switching to hen breeds that are better suited to non-cage housing.

The overall question is whether the original aims of putting hens in cages – to achieve better hygiene, lower disease occurrence and be labour-saving – remain a justification for limiting the birds' natural behaviours in a cramped space and denying them the opportunity for a good life. Enriched cages offer a possible solution, but space is still very limited and the hens' normal behaviour is restricted. Non-cage systems have the potential to offer laying hens a good life – which can be realized if they are well managed, for example with good hygiene and biosecurity – whereas cage systems, regardless of how well they are managed, do not. The view of the Federation of Veterinarians of Europe (FVE), representing the veterinary profession across Europe, together with the European Food

Safety Authority and many others, is that caging hens is no longer in keeping with our aspirations for ethically acceptable agriculture and that laying-hen welfare will be improved by moving away from enriched cages. FVE stresses that the necessary transition to higher-welfare systems should be done with appropriate care, minimizing known risks, but that in doing so hens should ultimately enjoy a good life, with both good health and a range of behavioural opportunities and positive experiences.

Other solutions include not eating eggs or, for those in a position to do so, keeping hens yourself, thus avoiding many of the problems intrinsic to large-scale commercial farming. When done knowledgeably, the potential exists to keep hens in small, stable groups with good health and opportunities for nesting, scratching, perching and foraging. Their inquisitive pecking around your feet is also quite endearing.

A bird lands on a nearby telegraph wire and begins singing as dusk draws in. A small, sparrow-sized bird of the countryside – a corn bunting – his chest visibly swelling as he raises his open beak towards the sky and scatters his jangling notes upon the evening air. He turns his head from side to side, listening for a response, ensuring no unwelcome neighbours have moved in since dawn.

The sun is now shining low across the plough lines over the field ahead. From beyond a long straight hedge that stretches to the distance, a white bird appears, flying slowly approximately two metres above the ground. Gleaming against the rich coal-black earth, passing through the silent space as a comet graces the heavens. The bird turns and banks vertically, disappearing into a grassy tussock. A barn owl's heart-shaped face is a floating parabolic reflector, hoovering the miniature patter of mice, voles and shrews from every crack, every depression, beneath every leaf. Every tiny footstep, every needle-thin exchange, escorted from the land via specially adapted facial muscles and channelled into waiting ears to ignite white lightning. The rodent victims see and hear nothing, but not every deadly strike is successful. The owl flies closer, talons empty, the streaming sunlight casting a halo around their pale wings as they pass close by, over the brook and beyond, with the composure and serenity of a cathedral bride.

The greatest friend to battery hens has been grocery shoppers. In fact, the rise in sales of free-range eggs over recent decades has become one of the most striking examples of the power of informed, concerned citizens in raising the standards of living conditions for farmed animals.

In 1998, just 21 per cent of eggs in the UK originated from non-cage housing systems. In 2008, this figure had doubled to 42 per cent and today it is 58 per cent. In response to this clear signal from citizens, major supermarkets have followed suit. In 2010, the first of the top supermarkets in the UK, Morrisons, announced that all of its boxed own-label eggs would become free-range, then in 2020 it became the first to extend this commitment to all eggs sold. In 2021, large food companies including Nestlé and Unilever wrote to the European Commission and European MEPs, asking them to phase out cages in animal farming, starting with enriched laying-hen cages. They emphasized that the business case for phasing out enriched cages is strong and noted that 'cage-free systems are widespread, economically viable, and provide better living conditions for hens'. Their timing coincided with a public hearing on the use of cages in farming (including for pigs, covered in Chapter 5) in the European

Parliament, triggered by an 'End the Cage Age' European Citizens' Initiative which gained 1.4 million signatures from across the EU. In response to this initiative, the European Commission, in 2021, committed to phase out cages in animal farming across the EU by 2027.

Countries outside the EU are also taking legislative steps to end the use of all cages for laying hens. Seven US states have enacted cage-free laws, resulting in over a quarter of eggs being produced in non-cage systems in the US for the first time in 2020. Moves are being made in Asia. In 2017 CP Foods, one of the world's biggest food companies, announced plans to phase out the use of battery cages for 100 per cent of the company's farms in Thailand, and a Cage-Free Egg China Summit was held in Shanghai in 2019. In 2016, Canada began a 20-year transition away from battery cages by 2036, though enriched cages will be permitted. In 2021, it was reported that Australia may phase out cages for hens, also by 2036.

On another issue – the killing of day-old male chicks – Germany banned the practice in 2022, followed by France. One alternative approach being trialled at commercial scale in Germany is to identify and destroy male embryos prior to hatching.

Each of these announcements cites shifting consumer awareness and pressure. Shopping is one of the most political activities we all participate in, and every time we exchange money for animal-derived products, we give our personal endorsement to the methods that produced them. Our purchasing choices influence how animals are reared.

As I had made my way up the long drive to the battery sheds on my first morning, I passed what looked to be free-range hens roaming in fields; I thought I must have reached the wrong farm. But they *were* free-range laying hens, and the farmer was clear in his explanation as to why they were there. 'I need to run a commercially viable enterprise,' he told me, 'and I know what percentage of my eggs will sell as free-range and what percentage will sell as caged.' In other words, as a business owner trying to make a living for his family, this farmer's choice of housing systems for his hens was not based on his own ethical priorities but on what will sell. And what will sell is, of course, determined by us. The farmer's approach was perfectly logical – if you pitch up at a market where nobody wants to buy chestnuts you will quickly go out of business as a chestnut seller.

People often ask me how they can make a difference to animal welfare. Where animal products are being bought and sold, ethical consumerism – the choices of informed, concerned citizens, all of us, in a free market – can be a powerful contributor to change.

CHAPTER 4

Sea cliffs and chickens

Llandudno Bay in North Wales curls gently into the seaside resort
of Llandudno, throwing ragged rocky fringes into the Irish Sea at its
extremities: the Great Orme, a hulking limestone headland to the west,
and the Little Orme, quieter and off the beaten track to the east. I had
visited the Ormes on many occasions during my childhood when my
grandparents lived in nearby Rhos-on-Sea. On this day, in the middle of
June, I was met off the train by my grandfather who dropped me at the
foot of the 140-metre Little Orme.

The weather is hot and sunny and I roll up my trouser legs before passing
through a kissing gate into the nature reserve. My trusty binoculars dangle
about my neck as I begin the ascent in the baking sunshine. A short while
later, passing through a leafy tunnel of overhanging warbler-filled scrub,
the path levels and opens out onto a limestone grassland plateau dotted
with linnet-topped gorse. A warm breeze blows on my face from the open
sea. Flecked against the dark waves, I see wheeling seabirds motoring
between the cliffs and their marine fishing grounds. June is the height of

their breeding season and seabird colonies are among the greatest wildlife spectacles in the British Isles.

It is midweek and I am alone upon the Orme. This is my favourite time to explore open spaces, when the rest of the world is engaged in its pursuit of productivity and I have hauled myself from the boiling rapids of everyday life. Up here I have transcended human civilization and passed into a timeless world of birds, butterflies and narcotic natural beauty. After scrabbling up a fissured rocky slope, I lie down flat on my belly on a slim grass-covered ledge and look out to sea.

To my left and right, 320 million-year-old cliffs plunge into foaming white waters. The geology is dizzying, as is the birdlife in the airspace ahead of me, where the endless toings and froings of fulmars, razorbills and guillemots whip entrancing spirals through the June haze. The razorbills and guillemots are auks, relatives of the well-known puffin. Like the puffin, they resemble small penguins in stature, with stumpy yet powerful wings that propel them effortlessly beneath the water in pursuit of fish. Such wings, perfect for their lives at sea (where they spend approximately nine months of the year) are barely capable of flight. The fulmars, on the other hand, are related to albatrosses. Superficially resembling gulls, they fly on long thin wings that barely bend in the middle, staying perfectly straight and board-like. This long narrow wing shape has minimal aerodynamic drag, perfectly equipping the fulmar to stay airborne on the slightest upcurrents, including those from the waves themselves. They take all but a few flaps in succession, then bank and glide effortlessly through battering storms and salty rainbows.

I watch a fulmar as they step from a cliff below out into a vast chasm of warm fish-scented air, then lift like a pantomime Peter Pan up through the echoing chamber of thousands of breeding seabirds. Six stiff, graceful wing movements push the bird away from the cliffs, where they connect with an invisible current and are flung far out over the sparkling sea, cutting through the sky like a fighter jet. They arc distantly within my binoculars, take five quick flaps, then sweep back towards the cliffs, now to my left, making minute, last-moment adjustments to negotiate the earth's jagged profile. The fulmar sweeps along the clifftop as though on a rail, their wings taut and unmoving, and flies past me, just metres away. After repeating the excursion three times, they make a final approach to the cliff, beat their wings more vigorously to brake and alight on the soft tussock. The bird chuckles and growls at their mate until they both eventually settle, their white plumage gleaming in the sunlight. Fulmars have some dark feathering around their eyes which gives them a gentle-natured look. The pair resume dozing and nestling in their corner of the seabird city.

Another seabird is present in abundance, forming a large breeding colony on Little Orme. The cormorant is a large black bird, ancient-looking, the closest one might expect to get to a pterodactyl. Found inland near lakes and rivers, as well as along the coast, cormorants dive to catch fish, then characteristically perch on rocks or waterside branches with their bedraggled prehistoric-looking wings held out straight either side of them to dry. Cormorants often fly low over water, interspersing slow wing beats with regular periods of gliding close to the waves, but now they are circling high above the sea in substantial numbers, soaring on the midsummer thermals and flying towards the cliffs.

From my grassy ledge I can hear cormorants honking and croaking beneath me. Wriggling snake-like on my belly, I cautiously edge forward, centimetre by centimetre, until the cliff face is revealed beneath me.

The whole sea cliff experience, already at a fever pitch of movement and sound, now builds to a crescendo of enmeshed criss-crossing flight paths, smells, cries, heat and the white froth of the breaking waves over a hundred metres below. The flooding of my senses rises exponentially the closer I shift towards the edge, my quest for more and more capped only by physical possibility. I feel as though the cliff could crumble away without consequence and I would be left spinning on the thermals, soaring down through the seabird colony like a fulmar, buffeted by the cacophonous growls and high whistling cries of my thousands of avian neighbours and flipped like a pinball around the crags and tussocks by the hysterical, repetitive 'kitt-ee-waaake, kitt-ee-waaake' screams of breeding kittiwakes. I feel drunk, intoxicated by this trance-like notion, then suddenly the sounds stop, fading away to nothing. Less than a metre beneath, a cormorant sits on their nest, cocking their head to look at me.

In everyday life a cormorant appears jet black, but at close range illuminated by the sun, the bird's feathers are metallic and iridescent, shining green, bronze and black with bluish tinges. The heavy, fish-catching bill joins bare reptilian skin on the face and this beams yellow on a clean white background. A continuation of this featherless skin between the cormorant's bill and neck billows rhythmically like a ship's mast in a breeze, a response to the stifling temperatures not unlike a dog's panting, called gular fluttering. The bird fixes their bead-like eye on me, and I, for a moment, fix mine on them. For a few short seconds I glimpse a bygone epoch and feel as though I have been plugged into the dawn of life itself.

Not wishing to disturb the cormorant, I retreat slowly from the cliff edge and stand up, pulling my collar back up around my neck to protect it from the intense sun. I continue walking along the clifftop in the direction of Llandudno Bay, then sit down again on the grass, looking out to sea, and pull a sandwich from my backpack.

Fulmar chicks produce a stinking oily substance in their stomach, which they regurgitate and spit at potential predators as a defence mechanism. On the islands of St Kilda, lying approximately 40 miles north-west of the Outer Hebrides in the Atlantic Ocean, a community of so-called 'bird people' once scaled the treacherous cliffs using ropes to harvest the fulmars and other seabirds who lived there. The fulmars' stomach oil was used as fuel and for medicinal purposes, their feathers for stuffing pillows and bedding, and gannet skins were used for shoes. The meat of all the harvested birds was also cooked and eaten. These hunter-gatherer communities lived on St Kilda, as well as Iceland and the Faroe Islands, until as recently as the 1930s when St Kilda was evacuated, and Iceland and the Faroes passed legislation banning the harvest of young fulmars due to their role in transmitting psittacosis (a bacterial disease) to the islanders.

The subsistence lifestyle of the St Kildan bird people, taking a seasonal product and drying it in hand-built stone shelters, contrasts sharply with the way bird meat is produced and consumed today. Given the numbers of birds involved, the title of 'bird people' might rightly now go to broiler farmers – those people across the globe who rear chickens for meat (broilers).

People often do not realize that hens kept for egg production and chickens reared for their meat are two different types of bird, farmed in different ways. Laying hens have been selectively bred for high egg production. Broilers, on the other hand, do not lay eggs but have been bred for rapid growth, so that in a short space of time their bodies comprise a great deal of muscle, which many people buy and eat as chicken meat. Broilers typically live their lives on the floor of a vast shed.

My first visit to a broiler farm was as unbelievable as I had come to expect from intensive animal farms. Despite, by this time, having visited a number of such places, I had still failed to fully anticipate and prepare for what I saw. From the outside, it was a long building situated close to a railway line and bordered by swaying crops. I was met by a farmer with a thick, check-patterned shirt and green wellington boots. He shook my hand with a grin, welcoming me warmly to his farm and, having kitted me out in a head-to-toe paper boiler suit and a disposable face mask, escorted me to the nearby broiler shed for my first exposure. He hauled a large sliding door to one side and I peered into the dark interior: a sprawling white sea comprising 10,000 jostling chickens.

A disinfectant footbath, to protect the birds from introduced pathogens, bubbled around my feet as the farmer and I entered the shed. I was at once engulfed by a cacophony of noise: loud, whirring sounds from ventilation fans in the roof space and a carpet of chirps and squeaks from the young birds themselves.

The farmer volunteered some information about the specifics of his enterprise: how he vaccinates his birds (via the drinking water), how many similar sheds he has on the farm (four) and so on. He then invited me to take as long as I wanted in the building while he returned to other jobs on the farm. The door slid shut behind him and I was left standing and staring at the birds stretching before me. Once my senses had adjusted, I stepped on to the soft floor, which was covered with a deep layer of wood shavings, and began walking slowly through the shed.

I walked the one hundred metres, from one end of the shed to the other, following the lines of feeders which ran the entire length. These gave rise to the constant tapping of chickens consuming unseemly quantities of ever-present grain. Similarly, long lines of suspended drinkers dispensed fresh water from nipples. As I penetrated deeper into the shed, as in the battery shed, I felt as though I had begun to journey into the centre of the earth itself. My familiar world became more distant and less accessible behind me, and I became a strange, erect loner among the swathes of shuffling chickens. Aside from the litter, the drinkers and the feed troughs, there was nothing but thousands of largely inactive birds. Today, in the UK, most broiler houses would additionally have straw bales, perches and pecking objects to promote interest and activity.

The domestic chicken is the most numerous bird on the planet. In the UK alone, around 1 billion chickens are slaughtered for meat every year, while the global figure is approximately 66 billion.

The simple lives of the birds who we may add to our shopping trolleys as chicken run broadly as follows. Fluffy yellow chicks (this is not intended to be sentimental, merely descriptive) hatch out from eggs in large incubators at a hatchery. At one day old the majority are transferred to a shed, such as the one I was standing in. They are tipped out of crates onto the soft wood shavings, where they begin to run about, peck and explore. The birds stay here like this, growing each day, for around 35–42 days, at which point they are removed from the shed and transported to a slaughterhouse. The shed is then cleaned and the next crop of chicks introduced for the process to begin again. When people learn of this rapid throughput of birds on broiler farms, they are often surprised to learn that most of the chicken meat we eat has come from birds who have lived for around six weeks.

The farmer describes his birds as well cared for and wanting for nothing. They have access to all the food and water they could ever want, are warm and dry at all times, and never at risk from predators such as foxes. So is this a humane farming system for producing vast quantities of protein for an ever-growing and hungry human world population?

We can identify a number of key challenges to the birds' health and wellbeing. The first, and arguably most important, is the speed at which these birds grow. In the 1950s a broiler chicken took 120 days to reach a body weight of 1.5 kilograms. Now, due to genetic selection, it takes just 30 days to reach exactly the same body weight. It is worth reminding ourselves that artificial genetic selection is a purely man-made phenomenon. This means, in crude terms, that when chicken breeders found birds who grew more quickly than the others, these birds were mated with each other. This meant that their offspring were also fast-growers. Among these fast-growing offspring, the breeders would then look for the birds who were growing the fastest and mate these together. These birds would then produce even faster-growing offspring and so on. Towards the end of their life, a modern-day broiler chicken can now put on up to 100 grams of weight every single day. The bird is effectively man-made: a creature who grows so quickly because of the way that their predecessors have been artificially selected and mated. When we find that such birds have health problems linked to their growth rate, it is we who have created those problems, as it is we who have created the birds themselves. Most would accept that it is therefore we who have a responsibility to correct them.

A key problem linked to fast growth is painful lameness, affecting millions of chickens globally. This can be caused by a range of possible diseases, which may be infectious (for example, caused by bacteria), developmental (meaning that the bird's bones develop abnormally as they grow) or degenerative (the bones or joints start to degenerate and become unhealthy, as in arthritis). Examples of infectious conditions include an infection that causes the top of the femur (the long leg bone) to die, while developmental conditions include those that cause the legs to grow bowed and deformed.

It is common to assess lameness in broiler chickens using a six-point scoring system, where zero is completely normal and five is an inability to stand. In a study that assessed the walking ability of 51,000 broilers in the UK, over a quarter (27.6 per cent) of the birds were moderately or severely lame (they had a locomotion score of three to five), with 3.3 per cent of these almost unable to walk. When applied to the total of 4.8 million birds represented (taken from 176 flocks), this means that nearly 160,000 birds were unable to take even a few steps. Over the last decade, breeding companies have increasingly selected against leg disorders and there have been improvements. Figures from Norway, for example, published in 2019, showed that 2.9 per cent of broilers were at the higher scores of four to five, compared to the previous 3.3 per cent figure. However, we should remember that even if this figure was at 1 per cent globally, this would equate to approximately 660 million birds being almost in too much pain to move.

To assess that pain, in a fascinating study published in the *Veterinary Record*, broiler chickens taken from typical farms (such as the one I was in) were trained to distinguish between different coloured feeds, one of which contained the painkilling drug carprofen. The University of Bristol researchers found that the walking ability of lame birds improved as they consumed more of the carprofen. In a second study, lame birds selected significantly more of the food containing carprofen than sound birds, and as the severity of the birds' lameness increased, the birds consumed a significantly higher proportion of the medicated food. People sometimes ask how we can know how animals are feeling. Experiments such as this, where animals are given the opportunity to self-medicate, lend compelling support to the hypothesis that lame chickens are experiencing pain. Additionally, and apart from the issue of pain, lame birds are also susceptible to suffer because of their inability to reach feeders and drinkers.

Another problem is the space available to the birds. When a sea of 10,000 chickens is seen for the first time, perhaps the most obvious initial concern is that they seem quite cramped, unable to freely stretch and walk about, the floor litter barely visible beneath a white blanket of wings, beaks and tails.

A high stocking density like this can cause a number of problems, not least that in their final weeks the birds are unable to move about and do the basic things that they would like to do and that would afford them a good life. As stocking density increases, so, in scientific studies, they are seen to jostle with one another more frequently and be more likely to be disturbed when attempting to rest. A normal degree of activity is necessary for healthy bones and joints, so as their activity decreases, more birds can begin to fall lame.

The rules determining how much space broiler chickens must have are described in terms of kilograms per square metre of floor space (bird weight per unit area). In 2000, the European Union's Scientific

Committee on Animal Health and Animal Welfare (SCAHAW) concluded that 'when stocking rates exceed approximately 30kg/m², it appears that welfare problems are likely to emerge regardless of indoor climate control capacity'. However, despite the SCAHAW's concerns regarding stocking rates higher than 30kg per square metre, a European Union Directive to lay down 'minimum rules for the protection of chickens kept for meat production' (which came into force in June 2010) permits a maximum stocking density of 42kg per square metre if specific measures are taken to control factors such as ventilation and temperature. UK government codes of practice permit stocking densities up to 39kg per square metre.

Following a substantial review, the European Food Safety Authority (EFSA) in 2023 recommended a substantial reduction in stocking density to a maximum 11kg per metre squared, to allow broiler chickens to express natural behaviour, to rest properly and to support their health.

Despite intensive broiler farming being, on the face of it, a fairly straightforward exercise of placing thousands of chicks in a building, letting them grow for six weeks then slaughtering them, life inside a broiler shed presents a suite of problems for the birds. Another key concern, highlighted by the European Food Safety Authority, is contact dermatitis, a painful skin condition, in which prolonged contact with the floor litter causes the skin to become red, inflamed and eroded, or, in severe cases, infected and ulcerated. The condition most commonly affects the breast, hocks (back of the legs) and feet, because it is these areas of skin that have most contact with the litter. Ammonia and moisture in the litter cause a type of chemical burn, leading to these lesions often being called 'breast blisters' or 'hock burns'. By now it will be apparent that many of the problems occurring in a broiler shed interact with each other, so in this case anything that causes the litter to become wet, or that causes the birds to have prolonged contact with the litter, will put them at risk of contact dermatitis. Examples of the latter include high stocking density (because of there being more faeces and the birds' movement being restricted) and lameness (because some birds are in too much pain to move and are more likely to sit down on the litter to reduce their activity). It would seem, then, that contact dermatitis, described by the EFSA as a 'widespread problem', is a further insult for millions of birds.

For broiler chicks to hatch out at a day old to be brought to a farm like this one, they must have come from an egg that was laid by a fertile parent. These birds are called broiler breeders. Broiler breeders also hatch at a hatchery, from where they are taken and placed in large single-sex flocks, typically comprising 2,500–3,000 birds. There can be several such flocks in a single house, so a broiler breeder house in EU countries typically contains approximately 10,000–30,000 birds. For the next 16–21 weeks, the rearing period, the birds simply eat and grow on a litter-covered floor. Then, at the onset of the production period, the single-sex flocks are moved to a different farm and the sexes mixed in a ratio of about one male to nine females. Until 60–65 weeks of age (that is, for just under a year) the males move around the shed, mating with the females who then lay fertilized eggs in nest boxes. These are then taken for hatching and the chicks are grown as the broilers previously described.

These broiler breeders are the birds who are producing the chickens that will reach two to three kilograms in around six weeks, so, predictably, these parent birds also reach high body weights in a short period if given plentiful access to food, like their offspring. However, with these parent birds the end goal is different. Unlike their offspring, who farmers want to be large and yielding plenty of breast meat, the requirement for the parents is that they are fertile and able to mate. Unfortunately, their high growth rate is compatible with neither; males that are too big, heavy or lame could not mount females and the fast-growing females often have abnormally functioning ovaries and poor fertility. To overcome these problems, broiler breeders are therefore prevented from feeding when they would choose to and kept continuously hungry. Instead of having unrestricted access to food to satisfy their ravenous appetite, the birds, during the rearing period, are fed a quarter to a third of what they would eat if given constant access to food.

When a stray, underweight animal, such as a dog, is found and given a meal, they can be seen to eat voraciously. Relating this to their own experience, most people have little problem in concluding that such a dog was hungry. The same, as would be expected, is seen in chickens, such that when their carefully measured portions of food are finally dispensed there is great enthusiasm to consume it and much visible competition between the birds to do so. At other times, these feed-restricted birds peck in their empty feeders and at the non-nutritive litter beneath their feet at a significantly higher rate than their non-feed-restricted counterparts elsewhere.

Another issue specific to breeder birds is distress and injury relating to mating. It may seem that there is nothing more natural than a male (of any species) copulating with a female to whom he is attracted. But sexual behaviour in broilers is described as 'rough', with males pecking and chasing females, and forcing them to mate. Females mated in this way may sustain feather damage and wounds to the back of their heads where the males have pecked and grabbed them, as well as to their bodies where the males' claws can rip their skin. Some people might say, 'Well if that's how chickens mate, that's how chickens mate, it must be natural for them,' but it should be remembered that under natural conditions (for example, in the jungle of their ancestors) females have the space and cover to escape from such aggressive or over-zealous males. In captivity, however, receiving unwanted sexual attention and associated injuries can become their way of life. Additionally, the behaviour may not actually be natural, as rough sexual behaviour and an absence of usual courtship may have been inadvertently selected for during the breeding programmes of broiler parents. In their reports on broiler breeder welfare, the EFSA suggest that genetic selection could be used to reduce the aggression displayed by many males during mating, together with reducing stocking density of the birds. Sadly, in a number of European countries, a more immediate 'solution' has been to subject the male birds to a number of mutilations, without anaesthetic or pain relief, at the hatchery, including beak trimming, de-toeing (removing one or more toes with a hot blade or hot wire) or de-spurring (removing the male's sharp claws, called spurs, by pressing them against a hot metal surface).

While reflecting on the injustice that we serve to billions of thinking and feeling chickens, my desire to see yet more of the seabird colony on the Orme grows and I want to view the spectacle from a different perspective. If I can get down to the base of the cliffs and around in front of them, I will be able to view them thundering towards the heavens before me, and watch the birds wheeling against the blue sky like a child's mobile. It would be the perspective that I had obtained on wildlife-watching boat trips in places like Skokholm and Skomer Islands in Pembrokeshire, and Noss in Shetland, but somehow I feel that I can achieve it on foot. The tide is out and I will simply have to paddle around.

I carefully make my way down the Llandudno Bay side of the Orme until I reach the rocky shore, then turn back on myself, leaving the pebbly beach for seaweed-covered boulders and rock pools. I must tread carefully and frequently steady myself as my walking boots struggle to maintain a grip on the slippery rocks. I can now see some of the birds on the cliff ledges above and I train my binoculars on these to watch their habits and interactions, but the main colony is still out of sight, just a little further round the seaward face of the Orme. The puddles are now starting to become more conjoined, until I am walking in an inch of seawater. I have walked sufficiently far that I can no longer see the beach behind me, but the promise of more seabirds pulls me dreamily and unthinkingly along the increasingly rocky and water-filled zone between the open sea and the looming cliffs. I give a thought to the potentially harmful effect of the salt water on my boots, as the water is now averaging a couple of inches in depth, so I remove them, tie them to my daypack and continue barefoot, clutching the slimy rocks as I go.

The seawater is now higher than my ankles and I am suddenly shaken from my addictive pursuit by a realization that the water is rising. In fact, not only is it rising, it is rising quickly and, as it progresses to the level of my calves, it becomes patently clear that the tide is advancing.

I am gripped by a sudden sense of panic. I turn around to look at the route I will need to retrace. What had been a landscape of water-filled craters in the shadow of the Orme is now a rippling blanket of lapping water and I begin to quicken my pace, fighting against the slippery rocks that pull my bare feet and legs sideways and backwards as I struggle to maintain my balance. The water is now at my waist, flushing waves of fear through me as great as I have ever experienced. I begin to crash and clamber through the cold water, feeling my feet and shins ripping against the sharp barnacle-encrusted rocks and the jagged shale beneath. The cold water rises past my belly button as I try to hold my precious binoculars above it and protect them from the salty splashes.

The incoming tide begins to seep through the base of my daypack and in the dragging surges, swallowed by the sea and removed from civilization, I feel vulnerable and worried. Then, as my limbs splash and crash, leaving feathery trails of blood rising up through the water in their wake, I suddenly feel the stable and relatively smooth surface of the pebbled beach underfoot. Overwhelmed with relief, I haul my wet body from the approaching tide like a turtle, stumble up the beach and collapse on a grassy bank at the top.

The experience scared me, and the bird identification guide that had lain at the base of my backpack remains wrinkled and tide-washed to this day. I had been reminded of the unforgiving nature of the world to which we belong and how, though I respect and adore it, all of us are equally insignificant in the face of its paths and patterns. Sometimes I have sought to watch wildlife at dusk, but left home too late to arrive in time. The dusk does not wait for me, it happens anyway. It happens in the way that it always happens, in the way that the waves always return to crash against the Orme. It is the way that, if global governments crawl slowly towards weak agreements on curbing anthropogenic greenhouse gas emissions, catastrophic climate change will happen anyway. The natural world does not wait or grant exemptions to its human inhabitants.

I had extricated myself from the powerful sea, but was still to learn how a sea of 10,000 chickens is successfully extricated from a broiler shed.

I was invited back to the broiler farm at 4:30am on a July morning. When I arrived, dawn had not yet broken and a lorry was parked outside the shed. I could hear clucking and flapping within and I entered the dark building to see men shuttling between a retreating tide of tightly packed birds and the shed door. The men were solidly built, like nightclub door staff, dressed in the obligatory paper boiler suits and white face masks. At the ends of their wide arms dangled flapping chickens, two suspended upside down by their legs from each hand. They were picked up from the floor, carried across the shed and placed into plastic crates on the waiting lorry, each crate taking 18–30 closely packed birds. Nobody said much to me, but I was encouraged to assist the catchers so I proceeded to pick the chickens up by their legs and make my own contribution to the depopulation effort. It was not long before my arms began to tremble with the burden of repeatedly carrying two birds in each hand, each weighing over two kilograms. The full-time catchers were essentially working as weightlifters.

One reason the birds were being caught at night was because, packed into crates on a lorry like this, temperatures rise rapidly and they become vulnerable to heat stress which can rapidly lead to death. Manual catching by teams of catchers is a common way of depopulating chicken sheds, but machines are also available for the job. These resemble combine harvesters, driven through the shed by a person, with rotating rubber fingers that scoop the chickens on to a conveyor belt, delivering them to the crates. Perhaps counterintuitively, studies suggest that mechanical catching may create less fear in the birds than the manual method I was assisting with.

The lorry drives from the farm, for as short a journey time as possible, to a slaughterhouse where the birds' short lives come to an end.

Is animal suffering an inevitable consequence of eating and enjoying chicken meat? If we are to rear and slaughter animals for food, it will never be entirely free from stress for the animals, but the key sources of suffering outlined for chickens here are neither inevitable nor unavoidable. However, addressing these problems will require a change in attitude towards chicken meat and the birds it comes from.

Most of the problems facing chickens reared for their meat are related to their fast growth rate and their impoverished living environment. Farming the birds in this way is a case of pile 'em high, sell 'em cheap. Despite there being thousands of birds, only a handful of stockpeople need to be employed to care for them. By utilizing all of the available space in the shed (by cramming the birds in at high densities and – in most countries outside the UK – not taking up any space with things that the birds might enjoy, such as straw bales), the greatest number of birds can be reared while minimizing all costs. By using fast-growing breeds, more batches of birds can be produced and sold in any given year.

The EFSA's Panel on Animal Health and Welfare stated that the broiler industry should have a strategic objective to reduce the high levels of lameness seen in broilers, 'even if this objective may require them to reduce growth rate'. Specifically, they recommend a maximum growth rate of 50 grams per day, down from the currently attainable 100 grams per day. Similarly, commenting on broiler breeder birds, it said that birds requiring less feed restriction should be bred from to address the problem of chronic hunger, 'even if this may involve [reducing ...] high growth rates'. So, just because we have bred these birds to grow as quickly as they do does not mean that such a trend, so incompatible with a good quality of life, should not and cannot be reversed.

Some systems of rearing broiler chickens are already seeking to minimize these kinds of welfare problems, namely free-range, organic and those under so-called 'higher-welfare' schemes, such as RSPCA Assured and Red Tractor Enhanced Welfare in the UK. In these systems, slower-growing strains of birds are used. Whereas a conventional broiler chicken will reach slaughter weight at just six weeks of age, free-range birds are typically slaughtered at eight weeks of age, while organic birds are typically slaughtered at twelve weeks of age.

Free-range and organic birds have the opportunity to access open space outside of their shed, with birds under Soil Association organic standards living in flocks of no more than 1,000 birds (compared to the 7,000–60,000 or so birds who may live in an intensive broiler shed).

Another important aspect of free-range, organic, RSPCA Assured and Red Tractor production systems is that the birds have something to do. Free-range and organic birds may perform their highly motivated behaviours, such as perching, scratching and dust bathing, on their range outdoors, while RSPCA Assured and Red Tractor birds, who may not always have access to the outdoors, are provided with so-called environmental enrichment: things such as the perches, ramps and straw bales mentioned earlier. These additions to the birds' environment increase the birds' activity which, in turn, improves their leg strength and reduces their risk of developing contact dermatitis. The number of animals, excluding fish, on RSPCA Assured farms has increased by 54 per cent since 2015, now making up about 11 per cent of the UK farming market.

Buying higher-welfare chicken is an action that individuals can take. Change can also come from retailers and food businesses making commitments on behalf of their customers. In the past three years, over 200 leading food companies – including KFC, Greggs and Nando's – have signed up to the Better Chicken Commitment, an NGO-led initiative requiring participating food businesses to meet specified minimum standards for broiler chickens by 1 January 2026. These include the use of slower-growing breeds and a maximum stocking density of 30kg per square metre. An independent commercial-scale trial investigating these two aspects of the commitment, published in 2020, confirmed that the slower-growing breeds had better health and experienced an improved quality of life through being able to perform a range of positive behaviours. Separately, a 2021 study found that slower-growing breeds require lower antibiotic use. Speaking about their signing up to the commitment, a KFC spokesperson said that people care now more than ever about the ethics of food production and that this is increasingly being expressed by their customers.

At least two things could help increase the market share of higher-welfare chicken. First is that all of us as citizens need to be aware of the consequences for chicken welfare, described in this chapter, that can arise from the commonest rearing practices. This should give us the desire to want to do something differently. Second is that we need to reset our perception of the cost of meat and other products from animals. Chicken meat is cheap because the animals are kept in ways that allow it to be so. It follows that improving their lives will require modest additional costs to be paid. In some cases, retailers and food businesses may absorb these costs. In others, there may be a modest increase in the cost of chicken that we buy, which may be less than many people think. People may be surprised to find that Britain's second largest retailer of RSPCA Assured products is the budget supermarket Aldi. Government support could help ensure these foods remain affordable to those on the lowest incomes.

Finally, we could also usefully look at the frequency with which food from animals is eaten. Chicken has shifted from being a valued food enjoyed on special occasions (for example, Sunday roast dinner) to something that is included in meals on many days every week. In 1950, British people typically ate less than a kilogram of chicken meat in a whole year; now we eat more than two kilograms every month. With no consequence for our nutrition and overall food budget, eating less chicken and paying a little more for it could spare hundreds of millions of birds the problems they currently endure on commercial broiler farms around the world.

CHAPTER 5

Orchids and pigs

The first time I saw a bee orchid was on a projector screen in a village hall. Stunning photographs revealed a plant whose flowers form exquisite three-dimensional replicas of visiting bees, and a local botanist embellished the flower's physical beauty with details of its equally fantastic biology. This flower was accessible to me and as soon as I heard about it there was no question that I must see one for myself. A week later I was in the dunes at Ainsdale National Nature Reserve on a hot June day hoping that I might find one.

I parked in the small dusty car park next to the Sands pub then gradually distanced myself from its cheerful summertime chatter as I joined a sandy track leading away from the beer garden and into the quiet dunes. My botanical knowledge is limited, but according to its website, the Ainsdale National Nature Reserve is home to over 450 species of flowering plant. On this day I was hoping to see just one of them.

Walking through the damp slacks, I soon found the lime-rich sand to be ablaze with carpets of flowering orchids. Many were early marsh orchids, but I trained my attention on the grassy margins around the damp depressions. Then, blowing gently in a warm coastal breeze, was a plant, approximately 30 centimetres tall, which threw intermittent, vivid mauve flowers out from a lanky stem. It was not alone; there was a small cluster in an area before me, all quivering slightly when the breeze picked up. In the quiet of the summer dunes the flowers bobbed and danced beneath the black and yellow furry bodies of their mounted insect mimics.

I dropped down on my knees and moved close to the nearest bee orchid so that I could examine its astonishing detail. The three mauve regular petals emanated from a single point out towards the corners of a triangle. Then, at the centre of these three, something remarkable happens. The orchid flower's lower lip is twisted and folded, manipulated by an invisible master origamist, until, at the centre of the mauve petals, rests a life-size furry bee. The petal bee model is incredibly life-like, decorated in extraordinary detail, with two perfectly formed antennae and a bee's velvety texture. The flowers were the culmination of between five and eight years' growth from seeds the size of dust particles.

The bee orchid is not the only orchid to craft its flowers into the shape of an insect; others in the *Ophrys* group of orchids do too. The names of the fly orchid and spider orchids, which can also be found in the UK, give clues to their petal creations. Via a mechanism of sexual deception and so-called pseudocopulation, these orchids have evolved to be sexually attractive to insects. Not only do the bee orchid's flowers resemble a bee physically, they also emit a sexually attractive perfume called a pheromone. The real bees land on the floral fakes and, as they attempt unproductively to mate with them, carefully positioned pollinia (clumps of pollen grains) adhere to the bee's back. Having left one flower, the bee is then deceived by the physical and chemical mimicry of another. Once again, the bee exerts itself in fruitless mating, transferring the pollinia and fertilizing this next orchid in the process. While such a mechanism is fascinating, bee orchids in their northern range (including the UK) have adapted to become self-fertilized. The reason for this is not entirely clear, but it has been suggested that the bee orchid's original insect pollinator may have become extinct in the UK following the last Ice Age.

If unthinking plants can evolve such means, it is perhaps unsurprising that humans, too, are prolific employers of inter-species pseudocopulation.

Humans artificially inseminate various animal species to ensure they can be bred according to our specifications. Certain domesticated animal species now exist in such a form that they persist through the act of artificial insemination – many are unable to reproduce by themselves – and people may be surprised to learn that the turkey, the culinary centrepiece of many Christmas and Thanksgiving celebrations, is one of them. Like broiler chickens, turkeys have been selectively bred for fast growth and large breast muscles which we can eat as meat. A wild male turkey weighs around 7 kilograms, but his domesticated counterpart can grow to weights in excess of 20 kilograms and, what is more, reaches this weight in around 20 weeks. By virtue of their exaggerated proportions these fast-growing birds are unable to mate naturally. The male is too big to get close to the female and, even if he tried, being much smaller and lighter, the female would be at risk of injury. Instead, to ensure production of most of the UK's 16 million turkeys (around 10 million of whom are eaten at Christmas time), workers are employed to manually milk semen from the male birds (stags, or toms in the USA) and then to inseminate the female birds (hens) with it.

Artificial insemination is also widely used in pig farming, and my first introduction was in a farm's small makeshift laboratory, when I stared down a microscope at wriggling pig sperm. The practice allows the sperm from desirable boars to be efficiently used to inseminate large numbers of sows, and breeding programmes have resulted in modern pig breeds with leaner meat and faster growth rates than their progenitors. The semen had come from a boar on the same farm and the farmer spoke proudly of the animal's productive attributes and genetic prowess.

Entering the farrowing house was quite unlike my first experiences of other farms, such as the caged hen and broiler sheds. Rather than the dim otherworldliness of those enterprises, the sliding door of the farrowing house opened into a brighter and more serene living space. Surreal, but nevertheless serene. For a start, the house was relatively bright, with small frosted glass windows admitting natural light. The house was not on the scale of poultry buildings, only around 20 metres in length, and from the entrance to the opposite wall was a long central walkway. Along its length, either side, were rows of 2-metre-wide pens, each containing a large sow with her litter of 10 piglets (the estimated EU average litter size is now around 14 piglets). The pens were low-sided, just a couple of feet high, giving an open-plan feel.

A radio quietly played chart music, which I was told was to accustom the pigs to the sound of human voices. Otherwise the building was quiet and undisturbed. You might expect 200 piglets with their mothers to create at least some gentle activity and movement, if not excitable play, but there was nothing. Just calm inactivity and occasional grunting from the sows. Why?

Aside from sows and young piglets being naturally quite restful, the pervading stillness was because closely surrounding each sow was a rigid metal frame. The sows were uniformly distributed throughout the building like carefully spaced allotment vegetables, each maintained at their permanent position by silver metal rails running beside their flanks and legs, and above their heads. The serene space was filled with scaffolding-like metal work, fixing regimented rows of mothers to a slatted floor.

The sows were confined in farrowing crates. Most people are now aware of cage systems for laying hens and, as we saw in Chapter 3, are increasingly expressing their disquiet or revulsion at the extreme confinement such cages impose, through their purchases and advocacy. But a similar degree of confinement in pigs is yet to fully penetrate the public consciousness. Bacon, sausages, ham, gammon, pork, Scotch eggs: these are foods enjoyed by millions and all derived from pigs, but all coupled with the likelihood of having come from animals subjected to months of rigid confinement, just like hens in cages, depending on the farming system they were raised in.

For many people, seeing inside a farm building populated with pigs in metal crates may simply be just that – a building populated with *pigs*: animals they can readily identify but perhaps less readily relate to or understand. They may have enough concern to be pleased that the sows have ready access to food and water, which those in crates do, but perhaps be less concerned that they are unable to move around, simply accepting that that must be the way pigs are kept. Worse, they may have preconceived notions that pigs are dirty or stupid when, in fact, pigs are neither. They have well-developed social and cognitive abilities, and normally use dedicated toileting areas well away from their resting areas.

Within a contraption that permits them only to stand up and lie down, it is not just their intelligence and desire for cleanliness that fail to be catered for. We have seen in Chapter 2 what would happen if the building was to deconstruct before my eyes; if the roof was to lift off, the pens to fall flat and the metal fingers of each crate to unfurl and release their stultifying grip from the pigs. Geography and climate permitting, and after an initial period of adjustment, the sows, like those in Stolba and Wood-Gush's Edinburgh Pig Park, would soon revert to the lifestyle of their ancestors, forming social groups with preferred individuals, spending hours rooting in the earth and tending to their piglets in nests they had diligently constructed one to two days before giving birth. Nest building is a highly motivated behaviour in sows and, as we saw in Chapter 2, in experiments it is performed even if they have been given a pre-formed nest of the type they would build for themselves. As a consequence, unable to do so, confined sows may be seen to become extremely restless, repeatedly trying to escape and rooting vigorously on the floor.

When pigs are viewed as 'just pigs' the building simply contains 'animals', kept clean, sheltered, fed and watered. But as knowledge of those animals increases, the farrowing house may be viewed as a great vacuum, powerfully extracting potential from its inhabitants: the potential of thinking, feeling animals and the lives they would prefer to be leading. It is populated by animals who want to do much but are able to do little. It becomes troubling and something which ought to be halted.

The sows living on this farm were among the nearly quarter of a million who live in this way at any one time in the United Kingdom. Pigs feature prominently on the planet's meat-eating landscape, with around a third of all meat consumed in the world being pork. The Food and Agriculture Organization of the United Nations estimates that there are around a billion domestic pigs worldwide, with around 143 million farmed in the European Union. In the UK, approximately 10 million are slaughtered each year, while approximately 409,000, like the sows on this farm, are kept for breeding. With such staggering numbers, it is clear that farming practices that compromise the welfare of pigs have the capacity to cause suffering for many millions of animals.

To help such practices to be considered, pig farming can be thought of in three distinct stages.

The first is the care and management of pregnant sows. The farm that I was visiting was a breeding herd, containing 420 breeding sows. Breeding sows are inseminated, pregnancy is usually confirmed using an ultrasound scanner (as used in humans) and, assuming all has gone to plan, they will be pregnant for an average of three months, three weeks and three days. Pregnant sows are called dry sows (because they are not yet producing milk for piglets), and how they are housed and managed is a distinct issue that needs to be considered when assessing the animal welfare impacts of modern pig production.

The second stage is the farrowing period: the time when the sow prepares for and gives birth, and then suckles her newly born piglets. This stage lasts for approximately a month.

At the end of the farrowing period the piglets are weaned, removed from their mother and mixed with other piglets in new accommodation. The piglets may initially be referred to as weaners and then, when they are a little older, as growing pigs, finishing pigs or simply growers. In this third and final stage the young pigs must simply grow each day until they are heavy enough to be slaughtered for their meat. This stage typically lasts for around three to six months, so that at four months of age they may be slaughtered for small meat joints or at six months of age for products such as bacon.

The sow will come back into heat and be inseminated five to seven days after weaning. She is then returned to the dry sow accommodation for the whole process to begin again. A breeding sow therefore has approximately two and a quarter litters each year and having had between around three to five litters (at around one to three years of age) the reproductive performance of many sows will diminish, at which point they are culled.

Back in the farrowing house, I was observing sows and piglets in the second of these stages – the farrowing period.

There is a reason why a mother is denied the opportunity to interact freely with her piglets or, indeed, to move about at all. Confining sows in crates allows more to be housed in each building, increasing the productivity of the farm business, and makes the sows easier to manage. In addition, farrowing crates have been developed to prevent the problem of sows unwittingly lying on, and crushing, their piglets. Paradoxically, this welfare insult to an intelligent and caring animal has arisen through a desire to protect her offspring from a different, serious welfare insult.

In the period between birth and when they are weaned, around 12 per cent of piglets born indoors will die in the UK. Causes include hypothermia, starvation and disease, but another important cause is when the sow of today's huge proportions lies down without realizing that her vulnerable piglets are beneath her.

It is argued that the farrowing crate is justified, therefore, on the grounds that it protects piglets from fatal crushing and suffocation. But is it? Is preventing *all* behaviour by the sow a proportionate response to the occurrence of one type of behaviour (crushing) that is undesirable? Economics and a desire to maintain maximum productivity has influenced the answer to this question in favour of the farrowing crate, but as awareness grows, consumers and citizens are increasingly unsettled about the consequences for the sows. We return to the driving ethical principle that all farmed animals deserve a good life, and systems are needed which achieve good welfare for both the sows and their piglets. The Federation of Veterinarians of Europe's view is that farrowing crates do not meet this crucial objective, stressing the 'urgent need' to move towards more ethically sustainable husbandry systems for sows and piglets. The International Veterinary Students' Association, the world's largest veterinary student association representing 40,000 members in 70 countries, publically backed the End the Cage Age European Citizens' Initiative and in 2021 urged the EU 'to phase out the use of farrowing crates in the shortest possible time frame and to promote a transition to well researched free-farrowing systems'.

Part of the solution takes us back to breeding and genetic selection. As pigs have been bred to be leaner and faster growing, breeding sows have become larger and clumsier. An unintended consequence has been a reduction in mothering ability. When genetic selection for improved piglet survival, rather than growth, has been examined, sows whose piglets survived well were ones who took greater care when lying down. It is necessary, therefore, for breeding programmes to focus on mothering ability in addition to productivity.

Another part of the solution is architectural, with research directed at designing farrowing accommodation that permits the sow to express her normal behaviour while offering protection for her piglets. So-called designed pens provide space and straw for the sow, but also incorporate features, such as rails or a sloped wall, to protect the piglets from crushing.

After two days on the pig farm, I was asked by the stockperson – a tall, boilersuit-clad man called Tom – if I wanted to assist with cutting the piglets' tails off.

We stepped into the farrowing house, walked the few metres to the nearest pen and sat down on the low barrier. A sow was lying in her crate, asleep, and ten two-day-old piglets were huddled on their nearby heat mat, also sound asleep. Prior to entering, Tom had filled a tail docking device with lighter fuel and he pulled it out of his pocket and lit it. After approximately two minutes, the cutting blade had reached its operating temperature of 400°C and he reached to pick up the first piglet in his large hand. Holding the piglet upside down and straightening their narrow tail between his fingers, he closed the knife across it, taking a couple of seconds to allow the high temperature to cauterise the blood vessels as it cut. By this time the piglet had woken up and Tom rapidly inverted the young animal through 180 degrees while reaching into his pocket for a second device. This time he pulled out a pair of stainless steel clippers and proceeded to hold the piglet's mouth open with one hand, while clipping the points off each of the piglet's four canine teeth with the other. He placed the piglet back in the pen, looked at me and grinned; 'Easy really, isn't it!'

I half watched the piglet tottering back to their littermates while half thinking how I might perform as a novice tasked with the same procedures. I had little time to dwell, as moments later Tom delivered a second warm piglet into my arms and I began to manipulate and reorient her while simultaneously getting a respectful feel for the red-hot tail docker. Seconds later I had burned my way through hair, skin, blood and nerves, leaving the piglet with a permanent stump in place of a tail and then, after clumsily removing the needle-points from the teeth, four freshly blunted tooth surfaces. This piglet then, too, tottered back to the group.

So far, so good, but by this time the whole litter had awoken and were on their feet. They squeaked and squealed as the mutilations continued to be executed ('mutilations' being not an emotive term, but the term applied to such procedures in British and European law) while their mother agitated through the sides of the crate. Tom continued docking and clipping rapidly and within a few minutes the procedures were complete, the excitement over and the piglets had returned to settle on their mat.

The justifications for such procedures were explained to me as follows. When litters are large or milk production less than optimal, competition for the sow's teats can be fierce. The piglets' needle-sharp canine teeth can cause injury both to the sow's udder and to the faces of their littermates, so they are blunted to minimize this potential damage.

Similarly, tail docking is also performed to prevent a perceived greater evil. Accommodation for growing pigs often lacks suitable material to forage and root in, so they may redirect their natural behaviour to the only available manipulable structures – the tails of other pigs. A tail bitten by other pigs can quickly be reduced to a bleeding stump, but, additionally, bacteria may enter the wounded tail, track up it and establish potentially life-threatening infection in the spinal cord. As well as the harmful effects on the pig, resulting abscesses can cause carcasses to lose value for the farmer. Tail docking is carried out to prevent the serious damage caused by tail biting.

We have seen, therefore, that three separate harms to pigs and piglets are inflicted to prevent the occurrence of different harms: farrowing crates to prevent piglet crushing, tooth clipping to prevent face and teat biting, and tail docking to prevent tail biting.

Some may argue that these mutilations are not painful. It should be recalled from Chapter 1 that pigs, like all mammals, have a nervous system similar to that of humans and are considered capable of generating pain similar to that which we experience. It comes as little surprise, then, that behavioural and physiological changes suggest that tooth clipping causes acute pain in piglets. Piglets who have had their teeth clipped are significantly more likely to display teeth champing (frequent opening and closing of the mouth), for example, compared to those who have only had their tail docked or only been handled. Clearly, the piglets appear to know that something has happened in their mouth. Additionally, histopathological evidence reveals that tooth clipping leaves the sensitive central pulp cavity open and exposed. The pulp cavity, as in humans, is the area in the centre of the tooth containing blood vessels and large nerves, and it is because of these large nerves that damage to the pulp can be extremely painful in people. As pigs have similar neuroanatomy and neurophysiology, it is highly likely to be so in piglets too.

It comes as little surprise that tail docking also results in signs indicative of acute pain. When piglets are mutilated in high numbers with speed and efficiency, each piglet is simply glanced at as they return to their littermates. But watched by trained observers for pain research, more subtle behaviours are detected. During and immediately after tail docking, these behaviours include tail wagging (intermittently flicking the tail from side to side or up and down) and tail jamming (clamping the tail stump between the hind limbs without side to side movement).

In addition, the researchers recorded a specific vocalization, called 'howling'. The piglets who howled were those having their tails docked. Most of the piglets struggled and vocalized intensely when they were picked up, indicating that they did not like being handled, but the only piglets that then howled were those having their tails removed.

It seems fairly self-evident that a piglet who howls and then wags or jams their tail stump is likely to be experiencing acute pain. But further evidence for the reliability of vocalizations as pain indicators is provided by studies looking at a third mutilation – castration.

Only around 2 per cent of piglets are castrated in the UK, because British pigs are slaughtered for meat at a relatively young age. But in other countries, pigs are older when they are slaughtered and as male pigs mature, their hormones cause compounds to accumulate in the fat which smell and taste unpleasant when the meat is cooked. This so-called boar taint is prevented by castration.

In many non-UK countries, therefore, piglets may not only have their tail and teeth cut, but also have their testicles removed with a blade at the same time. All of these mutilations are typically performed with neither an anaesthetic nor a painkiller being administered. In a Canadian study, researchers used microphones to record the vocalizations of piglets being castrated. Castration was associated with high-frequency calls, greater than 1,000 hertz. Pulling the testicles and severing their nerve-rich attachments resulted in more of these calls than the initial cut through the skin. A separate study showed that high-frequency vocalizations, as well as heart rate, were both significantly reduced when the testicles and supporting structures were first numbed with a local anaesthetic.

We can state with a high degree of confidence that tooth clipping, tail docking and castration are all painful. It is unclear how long this pain persists for, but an exposed pulp cavity can lead to painful abscesses and tooth fractures; and docked tail stumps often contain masses of nerve fibres called neuromas, which can be a source of significant and recurrent pain in people. What is more, this pain is being caused to large numbers of animals; it is currently an intrinsic aspect of modern pig production. The British pig industry reports that a 'high proportion' of indoor-kept piglets have their teeth clipped and that 72 per cent of pigs being reared for slaughter – affecting an estimated 7 million pigs per year – have their tails docked, despite routine docking being illegal. The UK has historically imported the majority of its pig meat and most non-British meat comes from pigs who have also had their teeth clipped and their tails docked, as well as being castrated.

Mutilations are painful and widespread, so it is clear that fresh approaches are urgently needed, which obviate the need for causing such widespread harm to animals who are providing us with food that many currently enjoy and value. The British Veterinary Association supports the UK Animal Welfare Committee's stance that 'sustainable agriculture should not depend on mutilations' and that the focus should be on preventing the need for such procedures.

As my time on the intensive pig farm came to an end, there was one final stage of the process that I was still to see. I had seen sows and piglets in the farrowing period and young pigs in the growing period. But once the piglets had been weaned and taken to the grower accommodation, what then happened to the sow?

Between five and seven days after her piglets are removed, the sow comes back in to heat and is once again mated or artificially inseminated. She is then moved to dry (pregnant) sow accommodation, where she lives throughout her pregnancy until, a few days before farrowing, the farmer returns her to another farrowing crate. Her life is one long cycle of pregnancy, suckling and being mated, as, indeed, it would have been for her wild ancestors. But life for these farmed pigs, as we have seen, is very different from the natural environment in which they evolved and remain largely adapted to.

On this farm, the dry sow accommodation was the least concerning of the pig habitations I was shown. Groups of around eight sows coexisted peacefully in modern well-constructed pens, loafing on beds of deep, clean straw for much of the time I spent watching them. When not nosing through the straw, they appeared carefree, finally able to move about and lie down where they chose. This is how many sows are housed for much of their nearly four-month pregnancy in the United Kingdom, but in some parts of the world their treatment following insemination may be profoundly inhumane and shocking.

In many countries, including most of the US, Canada and Brazil, many sows are moved from their farrowing crate to a separate building where, after insemination, they are placed in a metal contraption called a gestation crate or sow stall. Sow stalls are essentially the same as farrowing crates, but without space around them to accommodate piglets. Instead, the stalls form long rows, with each sow standing adjacent to the next, all facing forwards. These pregnant sows, like those in farrowing crates, can do nothing but stand up and lie down. They cannot turn round, dung away from their resting area or perform any of their natural rooting or exploratory behaviour. Housed this way, pregnant sows develop leg and joint weakness, and urinary tract infections linked to their chronic inactivity. Many are seen to become withdrawn and unresponsive – a condition known as learned helplessness, akin to clinical depression in people. Where activity *is* present, it is among those sows who have developed stereotypic behaviour, chewing incessantly at the metal bars before them or drooling frothy white saliva as they chew on nothing (so-called sham chewing). Stereotypic behaviours such as these are seen less frequently in the first few days of being placed in a stall, because during this period many sows spend their time trying to escape.

It might seem quite unbelievable that humans can place thinking, feeling animals like pigs in conditions as brutal as these, but the need to remain objective and focussed on rational argument is key. I watched a documentary in which a British presenter visited an intensive pig farm in the United States, where sows were living (existing) in stalls like these. The presenter asked the farmer whether he felt it was unfair to deny the pigs any opportunity to move about or do anything they might wish to do. His response was that the walk from stall to farrowing crate – a move from cage to cage that occurs approximately twice a year – constituted sufficient movement and that, while humans might not want to live in such a place, the pigs were content with their stalls. Essentially, he argued, pigs are not humans and we should not make the mistake of equating the experiences of the two.

As we so often see, this was probably not an uncompassionate or uncaring man, but someone who may genuinely feel that his animals' conditions were suitable. An alternative possibility is that he can see no other way to farm pigs profitably and has created a belief in his own mind that his system is suitable. Either way, if we are to argue against views like these we need to gather evidence – for example, of painful joint pathology and urinary tract infections, together with that from animal welfare science which identifies stereotypies and learned helplessness as indicators of hopelessly poor wellbeing. It is evidence of this kind that is moving arguments along and leading to improvements for the animals we keep and use.

My time at the pig farm eventually came to an end and I stepped out one last time, into the sunny farmyard and the chirping conversations of house sparrows perched on the gutters. Tom thanked me for the helping hand and checked I had gained what I needed. We discussed what I'd seen and he shared his own impressions of how pig farming was developing and changing. 'Times aren't easy,' he told me with an air of weariness. 'We're doing what's required of us, but our product isn't protected in the marketplace. We're being outcompeted for improving our standards and it doesn't make sense. It's not fair.'

He referred to changes in legislation intended to improve pig welfare in the UK but that he felt were impacting negatively on the British pig industry. Pigs in the UK, like elsewhere, experience suffering arising from several practices that have been described. In 1999, UK legislation was passed to end perhaps the worst welfare practice of all: that of housing pregnant sows in sow stalls. This should, of course, have been a significant step forward for the welfare of British pigs, but while the UK has banned this abusive husbandry system on its own soil, it has not been able to stop the import of pork products obtained from pigs housed using this same system elsewhere. In fact, to restrict trade on the grounds of differing animal welfare standards has been questionable under World Trade Organization rules, though this is now being actively scrutinized and challenged. Consequently, when faced with the two products – British versus imported – on supermarket shelves, uninformed citizens may tend towards the cheaper imported meat. Many would not do so if they knew the degree of suffering they were supporting with their purchase, but that information is not as widely available as it should be. Once again, and even with legislative progress, the role of citizens and retailers is key when considering the future of farmed animal welfare.

In 2008, nine years after the UK's total ban on sow stalls, the European Union passed a Directive that banned sow stalls across the entire EU from January 2013. Their use is still permitted for the first four weeks of pregnancy, but nevertheless, this was progress. As we saw in Chapter 3, in 2021, the European Commission committed to completely phasing out cages and crates in animal farming across the EU by 2027, responding to the will of citizens.

The US is also awakening to the mental and physical harm caused by stalls, with several states currently phasing out their use, and the same is happening in Australia. New Zealand banned sow stalls in 2015. Meanwhile, certain food-producing companies are voluntarily phasing them out in response to consumer pressure. Slowly but surely, the war against this particular source of pig suffering is gradually being won, but pressure will need to be maintained.

The 2008 EU Directive also legally requires that pigs receive 'enrichment' in their environment – for example, materials such as straw and hay which fulfil a pig's innate needs to root, chew, investigate and manipulate things – but the legislation is often ignored (with some countries providing nothing) or interpreted inadequately (such as the provision of dangling metal chains that soon become ignored). The Directive also prohibits tail docking from being performed routinely, but most countries illegally continue to do so, except some such as Finland, Norway, Sweden and Switzerland who have stopped routine tail docking and shown that it is possible to rear pigs with intact tails in commercial pig farming systems. There are repetitive infringements of the Directive in most EU member states, requiring national authorities to strengthen enforcement. If it is deemed by decision makers to be the will of citizens – all of us – further progress will be achieved.

June passed lazily into July. My summer of farm work was drawing to a close and I would soon get to take some holiday time with friends at home. But I had one more farm to spend time on and I left the north-west of England to experience life on a second pig farm in the south-east.

Pig farms can loosely be described as being either indoor or outdoor, depending on how the pigs are housed. Outdoor pig farming is more of a naturalistic approach, where the pigs spend some or all of their lives outdoors, behaving in ways that they choose. Farming pigs in this way requires low rainfall and well-draining land. Consequently, not all regions are suited to it, but the farm I was visiting had had pigs roaming freely on its chalky earth for 20 years.

I was staying with a university friend, Sarah. Starting at 7:30am, we emerged bleary-eyed from the house on Monday morning. The roads were quiet and soon Sarah's old Metro was motoring deep into the Sussex countryside.

Although early in the day, the temperature was already rising and we both had our windows fully down. High-sided hedgerows channelled us through the open landscape along pocked country lanes as we bumped past farm gates with aprons of cracked, baked mud and on towards a horizon of rolling fields and blue, cloudless sky.

We cautiously rounded a bend onto a long, ascending stretch of road. Occasional glimpses of the countryside below could be gleaned through the hedgerow, but as we neared the top, Sarah slowed and told me to look down.

Once again, as for all the farms I had visited, I felt as though I had fallen off the map, beneath the radar. Of the ten million pigs slaughtered in the UK each year, we barely ever see a single one. They are out here, in the managed wilds, away from our urban centres. As I looked down into the valley below, I felt as though I had been transported to Area 51. Stretching out across the land was a great, arid dust bowl dotted with currant-like black specks. Through the haze, and among the specks, pale rounded backs and lowered heads with large, flapping ears could be seen slowly shuffling between neatly spaced metallic shelters. There were 500 large sows roaming in 30 hectares of the British countryside.

Sarah turned a sharp left and began descending towards the farm. At the bottom, an inconspicuous painted sign revealed the farm's entrance and she dropped me off near an old, overgrown caravan and a large, corrugated machinery shed. As her Metro pulled away, the drone of a quad bike engine became audible from the opposite direction and moments later I was welcomed by a tanned, 50-something man with an unbuttoned checked shirt and a beaming grin. He introduced himself to me as Colin, the farmer.

'How are you doin'? Let's go in here, into the shade,' he said with a local accent, moving towards the corrugated building. Colin asked if I had had a good journey south, then began to outline the nature of his farm and how he manages his pigs.

If we recap the three stages of pig production – pregnant (dry) sows, farrowing sows and growing pigs – two of the stages, pregnancy and farrowing, took place on Colin's farm. Unlike the indoor pigs, the sows here are mated naturally by a boar. They then live in an outdoor paddock during their pregnancy until a week before farrowing, when they are moved to a farrowing paddock. When the piglets are born, they remain with their mother until four weeks of age, when, as in the indoor system, they are weaned. At this point, the apparent outdoor idyll ends for most piglets as they are loaded onto a trailer and driven to an intensive grower unit. Here, like the indoor-born piglets, they will live until they are of sufficient size to be slaughtered.

'Anyway, if you don't mind I'll leave you with Richard and he can show you how it all happens.'

I turned round to see a middle-aged man at the doorway, with rouge cheeks and wearing a drooping-brimmed hat. Richard nodded in my direction, then walked outside and hauled himself into the cab of a parked tractor. The engine jumped into life as he turned the key and he looked down at me expectantly. I pulled myself up into the cab and held on to a grubby rail as the vehicle set off with a jolt across the parched earth.

In a few minutes we had reached the edge of the dusty expanse that I had seen on the approach to the farm from Sarah's car. Richard idled the engine and jumped out to pull an electrified wire to one side. As he did so, a blanket of rooks lifted, fanning darkly on heavy wings and infusing the remote silence with harsh, agitated cawing.

Laid out in rows across the tinder-dry fields were corrugated stainless-steel shelters resembling miniature Nissen huts. They were called arcs and each one housed a sow with her litter of ten piglets. The arc incorporated a permanently open doorway, with a low grate surrounding the entrance to prevent the young piglets from escaping. The sow, however, could step out into the field as and when she wished.

Richard watched the sows for a few moments and seemed satisfied that they were healthy and feeding well. He started the tractor again and we resumed coasting slowly along the track, the movement generating a welcome breeze on my forehead.

The free-ranging sows also needed to keep cool as the morning temperatures rose. For this, each field had an excavated corner with water continuously pumped in from the nearby river. This turned the chalky soil into a pool of mud, and pigs strolled from their arcs to make use of the facilities. We pulled up next to a wallow and Richard stopped the engine.

It felt like a safari, stopping to observe the animals at their waterhole in the baking heat. A large sow stepped from the edge of the wallow and sunk down into the mud, which bubbled around her. She joined another who was lying motionless in the shallows with half of her body entirely submerged and her head resting on the side, her large ears drooped over her dozing eyes.

In my head I could hear the lyrics of the quirky, British 'Hippopotamus Song': 'Mud, mud, glorious mud. Nothing quite like it for cooling the blood...' With pigs being related to hippos, it was not entirely misplaced. The song's chirpy description of wallowing was accurate for both species, as pigs and hippos do not possess functional sweat glands so, instead, immerse their bodies in cool mud. Pigs, like humans, are prone to sunburn. When they leave their wallow, the mud smeared across their body dries and forms a protective layer against the sun's rays. The pigs I was watching were taking a dip in the pool and applying sunblock at the same time.

Richard jumped from the tractor cabin to the ground again, took off his hat and wiped it across his sweating face. He indicated that I should follow him and we walked in towards the nearest metal arc.

Within its shaded interior, a sow, dozing like her herd mates at the wallows, lay facing outwards. Her ten piglets were asleep within the hut and Richard reached in to gather them up. He had not explained why, but it quickly became apparent as he pulled a pair of stainless-steel clippers from his pocket and clipped the end off each piglet's tail. He visited the next few arcs for the same purpose, then ambled back to the tractor and transported us back from the suid wilds to human habitation.

It is fair to say that Richard was a man of few words and, having picked up a parcel of sandwiches, he disappeared into the caravan and closed the door. I had also brought some sandwiches with me, so retrieved these from the farm shed and took them outside.

I walked up the narrow farm lane with my sandwiches and climbed over a metal gate to enter a small field. The sun was now at its peak intensity and a large oak created a shaded refuge which I entered reverently. The air was cool and leafy, and I collapsed down onto the soft grass between the woody roots and began to eat.

The difference in lifestyles between the indoor and outdoor pigs had been stark. For the indoor sows, life shuttled between indoor pens and restrictive metal crates. The outdoor sows lived in large fields with a shelter in which to raise their piglets and the freedom to come and go as they pleased. The indoor sow was powerless to build a nest to protect her imminent litter, despite being highly motivated to do so. The outdoor sow gathered mouthfuls of straw and carefully arranged it in accordance with her powerful maternal drive. Without good management and stockpersonship, the outdoor sow would be vulnerable to extremes of temperature in summer and winter, but on this farm her needs were diligently catered for, with well-designed shelters and straw replaced weekly in the summer and twice weekly in the winter. As I had seen for myself, cooling wallows were optimally maintained and well utilized by the hot animals.

The young piglets on both farms had their tails docked. This was deemed necessary because both indoor and outdoor-born piglets were transported to indoor grower accommodation after weaning, where the barren pens and lack of environmental stimulation increased their risk of having their tails bitten. A high proportion of indoor-born piglets have their teeth clipped, but for outdoor-born piglets the proportion is generally lower.

As I sat reflecting, I had gradually become aware of a commotion from a flock of jackdaws in the branches above. Listening to their exclamations, I thought of the Nobel prize-winning ethologist Konrad Lorenz, whose book *King Solomon's Ring* describes his observations and affections for a colony of tame jackdaws around his Viennese home, including how the birds culturally transmit information about potential predators from one generation to the next. Lorenz noted a particularly vehement 'rattling reaction' that expresses, 'even to the human ear, the emotion of embittered rage'. I turned to see if I could see what was happening, forensically scrutinizing the branches through the green stained-glass windows of the oak's canopy.

My gaze locked onto two singular black points surrounded by blazing yellow halos. A pair of piercing eyes sent their burning fire into mine from deep within a fierce frown. The source of the jackdaws' disquiet was a little owl who bobbed their head up and down while maintaining their unflinching gaze as they tried to gather information about the unusual visitor sitting beneath their tree. Little owls are the smallest of the UK's owls and the most likely to be active during daytime. I held my breath as I looked back at the beautiful owl for a few seconds longer, before the owl turned and launched themselves out in to the sunny countryside. A few seconds later, the jackdaw colony also lifted from the tree, dispersed into the bright sky above and left me sitting alone in the quiet once more.

If consumers of pig-derived products feel that the lives afforded to some of our pigs are unacceptable, they can choose to avoid them completely or support higher-welfare farming systems through their shopping purchases. Currently, around 40 per cent of breeding sows in the UK live outdoors and give birth to their piglets in arcs, while most of the remaining 60 per cent are locked into farrowing crates during this time.

Almost all (around 96 per cent) of their offspring, the growing pigs, are housed indoors after weaning, even if, as on this farm, they have been born outdoors. Only 3–4 per cent of growing pigs spend their whole life outdoors before being taken for slaughter.

Unlike the rules relating to egg production, there are currently no legal definitions of terms such as 'free range' when they are applied to pig production, and this has created confusion for UK shoppers wanting to support improved pig welfare. The meanings of some common terms currently used on pig product labels are as follows.

- **Outdoor bred**: The sows live outdoors in an arc and are able to build a nest for their piglets. At weaning (four weeks of age), the young pigs are then moved indoors where they live until they are slaughtered. The indoor system may be straw-based (for example, if they are RSPCA Assured, see below), otherwise the pigs may be housed on slatted or concrete floors. Products coming from the pigs born on the outdoor farm I visited would be labelled as outdoor bred.

- **Outdoor reared**: The piglets are born outdoors, as for outdoor-bred piglets. But rather than the young pigs then being moved indoors at weaning, they are moved to outdoor pens instead. They spend around half of their life in the outdoor pen, then they are moved indoors, where they live until they are slaughtered.

- **RSPCA Assured**: RSPCA Assured pigs may live indoors or outdoors, but their living environment is monitored according to strict welfare standards. They must always be given straw to root in and they are given more space in which to exercise, play and rest. The use of farrowing crates is not permitted and tail docking is only permitted in exceptional cases.

- **Free range:** Free-range pigs are born outdoors, then should spend their entire life outside in a field with arcs to shelter in. Sows spend their life outdoors. Farrowing crates are not permitted and tail docking is typically not needed.

- **Organic:** Both sows and piglets are kept outdoors for all their lives. Farrowing crates are not permitted and tail docking is prohibited.

Buying pig products carrying one or more of these labels can be a positive choice for animal welfare, because these systems confer welfare advantages to the sow, growing pigs or both. If a pig-derived product, such as pork or bacon, does not carry one of these labels, then it has probably come from animals reared intensively indoors. Well-managed outdoor systems planted with trees and other vegetation may also form part of agroforestry approaches, currently being explored to achieve climate change, ecological and animal welfare objectives.

A note can be added about organic pig production. Organic production puts an emphasis on the essential aspects of good stockpersonship and management, alongside judicious use of permitted medicines. The use of conventional medicines is restricted. Health problems can affect animals in both organic and non-organic farming systems, with a comprehensive review published in 2021 concluding that neither one nor the other currently performs better on overall health status. Organic systems offer greater opportunity to perform highly motivated behaviours, which is central to an animal's prospect of enjoying a good life, so offer good welfare potential. For this potential to be realized, disease prevention and treatment must be afforded the same high priority it requires in all systems.

Some people feel that buying pork products of British origin is the way to support higher standards of pig welfare. As was noted earlier in this chapter, Britain banned sow stalls in 1999 and British piglets are not castrated. But it remains a fact that nearly 60 per cent of sows in the UK give birth in farrowing crates. Looking for the Union flag and Red Tractor assurance scheme logo on pork packets can be a step in the right direction, but standards under this scheme go little beyond minimum legal standards. Simply buying British, without also looking for one or more of the terms listed above, will not yet provide a solution for the other important animal welfare concerns outlined in this chapter.

There is currently a once-in-a-generation opportunity to improve pig welfare in England, including ending the use of farrowing crates, with the UK government's Animal Health and Welfare Pathway, which is in development. Following the UK's departure from the European Union, many organizations, including the British Veterinary Association, successfully lobbied for post-Brexit domestic agricultural policy to be based on 'public money for public goods'. This policy aims to reward farmers with tax-payers' money for achieving high standards of environmental stewardship and high animal welfare. Now, the details of how that additional money might be spent are being planned, including proposals to support progress on tail docking and moving to non-crated farrowing systems. Meanwhile, in progress elsewhere, the New Zealand High Court, following a highly contested legal challenge, ruled in 2020 that the use of farrowing crates is unlawful under New Zealand's Animal Welfare Act.

CHAPTER 6

Goose days

The days began to shorten and the temperature cooled. I had enjoyed visiting sparsely populated regions of the British countryside, but less so seeing, first-hand, how some of our most intensively reared farmed animals must live their lives.

During my short summer break, I returned to my home in the north-west of England. As September drew closer, the advancing autumn tightened its grip on each passing day. Occasional gold tinting began to glint from the tops of deciduous canopies, gradually spreading from one to the next. Within weeks, the woodlands were gleaming bronze, copper and gold, as clusters of exhausted leaves danced jubilantly on the autumn breezes until they dropped.

A thousand miles away, in Iceland, the glowing British Isles are in the sights of half a million pink-footed geese. When September finally arrives, these birds lift from the tundra, where many have raised goslings over the summer, and set airborne armadas on a course towards Britain's beacons. Despite having been fortunate to experience a number of wild spectacles across the world, the sight and sound of the returning geese is still, for me, the most affecting of them all. South-west Lancashire is visited by 40,000 or so pink-feet, who divide their time between the agricultural mosslands inland of Southport and Formby, and their evening roosts on the estuaries of the rivers Ribble and Alt, and at the Wildfowl and Wetlands Trust nature reserve at Martin Mere. Formby lies beneath their flight paths to and from these winter locations and I would typically hear my first geese of the year flying above my parents' home at night. Their arrival seems as certain as the falling leaves and, having heard them every autumn since I was a young child, my ears are attuned to their 'wink wink' calls passing overhead. Even now, I must immediately stop what I am doing when I hear this call and race to the nearest window or out through an open door to crane my neck skyward. Against the dark sky, I am just able to make out the movement and silhouettes of birds flying on shallow wing beats in the direction of the coast, their occasional calls in the quiet night air gluing straggly groups together.

Over the coming months, the diurnal rhythms of the geese travelling between their estuarine roosts and farmland feeding grounds become a feature of the local landscape. Their dark airborne squadrons are seen when out driving, or passing over central Formby at dusk, where shoppers can be seen to stop and look up at the sky. At night, groups may be quite quiet in flight, calling only intermittently, but at dusk the passing geese arouse attention. Their size and thousands-strong numbers make them highly visible and they call constantly to maintain contact with related birds, while ensuring their ranks remain in characteristic V-formation.

Their daily movements swing like a metronome from the rising to setting sun, so the most reliable sightings of the geese in their greatest numbers are frequently linked to dramatic winter skies. For my first dawn encounter of the year, I waited for a sunny forecast and then made my way to the Alt Estuary before first light, where it is not uncommon for around 10,000 pink-footed geese to spend the freezing winter nights.

I park close to Blundellsands Sailing Club and step out from my heated car into the dark, cold air. The silhouetted roofs of nearby houses stand quietly beyond the boat yard's tall masts, their trussed rigging clinking rhythmically in a gentle wind coming up the river. I put on my hat and gloves, zip my jacket up to my chin and set off on a sandy footpath leading alongside the muddy channels of the Alt and into the pale dunes.

After a short walk, the path bears to the left, opening onto an apron of sandy beach. The dunes with their covering of spiky marram are now behind me, with the sleeping village of Hightown just visible beyond. To the south, eight miles along the coast, the lights of the port of Liverpool twinkle through the morning mist. Stretching out ahead, and sweeping round to the coastline either side, are the dark mudflats, which run into the Mersey Estuary and Liverpool Bay. Facing out towards the distant water, I can hear the low crashing of the Irish Sea and occasionally, when the wind blows in my direction, the squeaking calls of pink-footed geese. They are out there, in the darkness. I shuffle my feet on the cold, hard sand to encourage circulation and clench my numbing fingers within my gloves.

The geese find their nightly refuge within a bleak landscape. I raise my binoculars towards the shoreline, sweeping them past water channels carved in the mud and the meandering Alt itself, dotted with buoys and marker posts. Low fog swirls above the watery channels and far beyond, where the choppy tide meets the squelching land, I can see a slim dark band running along the water's edge. Straining my eyes in the dim light, I see that it comprises individual geese standing in the waves and on the soft mud. They are isolated, safe from predators and human disturbance as they require. The line of geese stretches as far as I can see, before becoming indistinguishable from the murky waves rising and falling behind them.

Over the minutes that follow, my tension and anticipation rise with the climbing sun. As the sky gradually brightens, a pale orange band appears low across the eastern horizon and the warming sun begins to burn off the morning mist. I can still hear the geese out on the estuary, but their activity is linked to the breaking dawn and their calls are reaching me more persistently. Now, rather than the sound blowing on occasional gusts, I can hear it constantly, the rabble growing in intensity.

The building commotion indicates their imminent departure. Then suddenly, with an energy like the raging sun itself, the simultaneous calls of thousands of wild geese become clamorous, reaching a peak as though the whole landscape has been sucked within a giant metal drum in which the geese fill my mind with a noise that is echoey, tinny and deafening. With it, the geese lift from the mudflats as a dark haphazard mass and begin flying towards the beach where I am standing. The scene is all-consuming and, having waited in the biting morning air for this single moment, I struggle to know where to look as the advancing geese assemble themselves into their structured V-shapes and spread out in long trailing lines, calling constantly. Their reflections start appearing in the still waters of the Alt just ahead of me, their arrowhead formations now flying towards the risen sun and their lacy skeins stretching far into the distance, north and south, against a collage of feathery orange clouds.

They fly above my head, over the misty dunes, and as their calls fade into the wakening day, they disappear towards the fields where they will spend the day feeding.

Moments later, a second huge group take to the air, repeating the scenes of the first. Over the course of a quarter of an hour or so, several skeins of varying sizes leave the roost, all departing in the same direction towards the mosslands. Exhausted by their relentless beauty, I look back out to sea and can see no more geese at the water's edge. There is some relief in the thought of returning to the shelter of my car and home to a warming bowl of porridge.

In the final weeks of my time at home, my parents had been receiving an unusual garden visitor. A fox cub in itself wasn't especially unusual, although we rarely saw one, but one that seemed confident and unperturbed by humans was quite unusual and afforded unique and intimate moments.

The first encounter had been in July. I was upstairs and heard my dad calling my name in an urgent whisper. I ran downstairs to find him standing still at the open front door; he turned slowly towards me and beckoned me with a small hand movement. I quietly joined him at the doorway and looked out. A short distance along the front path, a young fox cub was nosing around the flower bed. His fur shone ginger in the late afternoon light and, as we held our breath, he proceeded along the path towards us, stepped onto the lawn and crossed a few metres in front of us. As he disappeared into the leafy beech hedge, my dad and I turned to look at each other with a shared feeling that we had had a special and memorable sighting.

A month later the small fox appeared again. Again in daylight and this time in the back garden. Bright, inquisitive eyes beamed from beneath alert, oversized ears and he was relaxed, trotting and sniffing around the grass. Something about his posture and movements signalled playfulness and mischief, and this time I stepped outside into the back garden to see if I could get a closer view.

The cub stopped what he was doing and leant forwards with his cavernous bushy ears angled towards me. He looked at me with twinkling eyes, then turned and skipped down the garden. But he didn't run with terror. Instead he stopped at a flower bed, flopped down onto the grass and lay looking at me, his tongue lolling from an excited mouth.

It was clear that the fox's attitude towards people was not what you might expect and that he seemed to view the presence of humans as interesting and engaging rather than frightening. I went back into the house and returned with a packet of ham. (Following on from Chapter 5, I would always advocate sourcing ham with one of the higher-welfare packet labels.) Lying on the grass, I tore some thin strips of the meat and threw them out in front of me.

The cub rose to his feet and started walking towards me. He was a bit more cautious this time and he lowered his nose to the ground, keeping his ears firmly fixed in my direction. He looked up frequently and then found the first scrap, licked it up and quickly swallowed it. The cub remained relaxed and moved further towards me with his nose lowered to the ground. It was sunny and he was now within three feet. I was enjoying the animal's company; regardless of how people feel about foxes, no one could fail to be impressed by this creature's beauty. His coat was a warm gingery-orange with a thick pile of faintly pale-tinted, well-groomed hairs sleeked from head to toe. The backs of his ears were black, meeting burnt orange fur glowing at their base. Two black bands also slipped away from the bridge of his nose and down the side of his long muzzle, first across the orange baize and then meeting a clean white strip which ran away from his jet black nose tip, down his neck and towards his chest. Each of his four limbs became a darkened continuation of his ginger flanks, culminating in black socks and paws, with the trademark thick auburn brush trailing behind. His markings were quite exquisite.

The cub finished the last of the scraps and looked at me. I put a piece of the tacky ham on the end of my fingers and lay my outstretched hand flat on the ground. He paused, stepped forward and next I felt the soft fur around the end of his nose brushing against my fingers. We exchanged several glances, but as soon as I shifted my position he skipped back down the garden and lay down next to the flower bed.

This ham-focussed relationship continued for the next fortnight and during this period I began to announce my arrival with a 'hoo-oo, hoo-oo' call. The cub seemed to spend his time relaxing in the shrubbery around the garden and soon I had only to step outside, and with a 'hoo-oo', there would be a rustle in the undergrowth and my new companion would emerge onto the lawn.

After a while, he began to value more than just food. I had a yellow tennis ball on a length of a cord and took it with me one day. He found it fascinating and proceeded to pounce on it and bat it with his paws. He also felt my shoelaces were fair game and often tried to sneak up behind me when I was sitting on the lawn and undo them with his mouth. If he was caught in the act he would jump away playfully, then as soon as my back was turned, would jump forward and I would feel tugging at my feet once more. These games progressed, until we were both playing on our feet. I would pretend to jump towards him, causing him to bounce back, and then he would spring forward, causing me to side step and turn. One evening, frisking like this on the grass, we ended up close to a wide-based conifer tree in the garden and I pretended to pursue him. He turned and ran, but only as far as the other side of the tree. Peering through the thick branches, I could see him looking to see where I was and I quietly crept around the side of the tree. Then, when I jumped out to surprise him, the dusky garden filled with silent laughter as he raced around to the other side of the tree. If I went left, he went right; if I went right, he went left. At any time he could have run away with fear and never come back, but the game continued for many minutes: round and round the mulberry bush, as you would play with a young child or a domestic dog. Neither of us had been taught how to play this game, it was entirely spontaneous, but we both knew the rules and we raced about the bush until darkness fell and we were tired.

Quite why the young fox cub had arrived tame at our garden was a mystery, but any animal's behaviour is a result of the interaction between their genes and life experience. Perhaps the cub had simply been born with a bold temperament. Perhaps he had had close, positive contact with a human or humans at a very young age, though it is hard to imagine why or where. If he had been rescued, it would be unlikely that any responsible wildlife rescuer would release a tame, and possibly human-dependent, fox into the wild to fend for himself, though perhaps he was tamer than they realized. But whatever the reason, he was here and in good physical condition, obviously finding more to eat than scraps of ham, and enjoying playing games in our garden.

The close interaction we were having also gave me interesting insights into aspects of the fox's psychology. He seemed to be an animal who wanted to identify the source of things that he valued or found appealing. Playing with the tennis ball on the end of the cord was fun, but trying to steal the cord at its origin was even more so. Whenever he took ham scraps, I noticed that he would always be spying the packet at my side from which they came. The scraps were keenly accepted, but you could see that he felt having the packet would be even more worthwhile. As he became more confident around me, he tried to approach the packet several times, despite being freely offered small pieces, and on one occasion snuck in beside me and managed to drag it away in his mouth. The behaviour reminded me of a habit that foxes are well known for, and which contributes to their poor reputation among some. Foxes have an infamous relationship with chickens and can wriggle through impossible fence gaps at night to access the sleeping birds in their coop. When they do, they invariably don't just take one of the birds, which could provide a satisfying meal, but apparently wreak havoc in the henhouse, embarking on a killing frenzy that can leave all of the birds slaughtered. Why?

It is not because the fox is 'killing for fun', as some people claim. Entering the coop is extremely risky for the fox and, as they do, they may be quite fearful as they become enclosed within a space from which they cannot quickly escape. But their hunger, or that of their waiting cubs, spurs them on. Once inside, they are faced by a situation that would have been unusual during their evolutionary history. Rather than their skills of prey detection and problem solving leading them to, say, a ground-nesting bird, perhaps with a clutch of offspring, as would have been the case with their ancestors, the fox entering the world of domesticated livestock is suddenly faced by potentially hundreds, if not thousands, of possible meals, repeatedly triggering their predatory behaviour. Then, having expended energy and taken a risk, foxes have evolved to perform caching behaviour, where they move the surplus carcasses to a number of hiding places for future consumption.

When the prey is a chicken, they can usually drag only one away in their mouth at a time. When a fox enters a henhouse and engages in such surplus killing, they are then either unable to drag and cache *all* of the birds (because there are simply too many), or, while removing some, they are disturbed and flee, leaving the others behind. Either way, the next human to attend is met with a scene of apparently wanton carnage and when that person is the hens' caregiver, the red fur snagged on a wire fence is enough to deeply test their tolerance of foxes. The fox, however, has simply acted in accordance with behavioural tendencies evolved over millennia, which, outside of their control, misfire in the face of high populations of domesticated animals in the modern world.

Before the summer was over and a new university term began, I arranged, with three former school friends, to take a boat trip to Norway. The mini-cruise departed from Newcastle at 7pm on 1 September, calling at Bergen on the evening of 2 September and then returning to Newcastle on 4 September. When we weren't on land, which was all the time apart from the evening in Bergen, we were passing slowly up the Norwegian coastline or crossing the open waters of the North Sea.

We said goodbye to the port at Newcastle beneath a dark pink autumn sky and soon had the sea wind blowing on our faces, as terns jinked and dipped on the gusts and dark cormorants flew overhead towards the land. An Arctic skua, known for their thieving and bullying, could be seen harrying a gull ahead of the boat, banking left then right in pursuit, with a single piratical intent of doggedly wearing the gull down until they surrendered their meal. When we arrived at Bergen, heavy rain lashed past the lights on the harbour side, and we disembarked with our collars turned up to the elements and made a dash for the nearest bar. At 2am the socializing and sea air finally got the better of us and we retired wearily to our cabins and sunk into our bunks.

Four hours later, I was awoken by the piercing beeping of my alarm. I was shattered, but had wanted to rise at dawn at least once during our trip. My friend rolled onto his other side without waking and I stepped out into the boat's narrow corridor and quietly closed the door behind me.

I heaved open a solid metal exit door, admitting a rush of salt air from a cloudless hazy peach sky. The empty deck glistened with salt spray and I leaned against the safety rail with the fresh morning wind blowing on my face and looked out across the motionless water, the stillest and calmest I had ever seen.

Off the starboard side, something cut through the silky drape of the water and momentarily emerged into the dawn air. The absence of waves meant that I could see anything on the sea for miles around, and I had already seen guillemots rafting on the surface and a diver (a type of seabird) on the water in the distance. But this was different and closer. Curved like a sickle and black. Arched then vanishing. I was sure I had seen a fin.

Now I was fully awake, adrenaline pumping through my body and my heart banging in my chest. I clutched the rail and scoured the water with obsessed, unblinking eyes. I had never seen a whale or dolphin before and I knew that sightings in the North Sea were possible. Then, a few metres to the right, it happened again, real and unmistakeable. I was watching a whale.

About the same length of time passed before the whale surfaced for a third time. Their dark arched back and erect dorsal fin was the only visible protrusion above the glassy water for miles around and I felt my mind expanding impossibly. I had to share my sighting with someone and, running as safely as I could without slipping, I clattered down the metal steps, along the corridor and burst into my bedroom.

'Mark!' I whispered loudly. 'Mark!' My friend stirred and looked at me. 'There's a whale!'

He didn't need telling twice. He threw clothes on quickly and followed me, running back along the corridor and up onto the deck. The sun had now appeared fully from beyond the horizon and greeted him as a shimmering golden disc reflecting in the sea. Beneath it, the dark minke whale surfaced again before making a final dive and disappearing for good. Mark and I grinned at one another like delighted children.

We stayed on deck for the next three hours, seeing a school of dolphins bouncing in unison across the open sea and gannets gliding above the boat. Seabirds have adapted physiologically to cope with storms and bitter temperatures, but seeing them hang in the blank sky above the endless water I was reminded of their behavioural adaptations which make such a life seem normal to them. These varied and sometimes alien environments in which species have evolved are what we must bear in mind when designing environments for captive animals, including those who are domesticated, to meet their behavioural needs, protect them from stress and frustration, and help ensure their captive lives are good ones.

When I returned to Formby I was keen to catch up with the young fox. I stepped outside and issued my familiar 'hoo-oo' greeting, but there was no response and eventually I went to bed wondering what might have become of him. This was repeated over several nights and I began to suspect the worst. Then, one evening at 10:30, after an absence of two weeks, I looked outside to see a fox in the dark, on the lawn. I couldn't be sure, but I dared to imagine it was 'our' fox and went outside. The animal was visibly larger, looking more like an adult than a youngster, but when I sat down he started slowly walking towards me, paused, and then stepped forward to take ham from my hand. My companion had returned.

As he had matured he had become more nocturnal in his ways and typically arrived in the garden at dusk or later. We continued with our nightly games of chase and he had developed a clear way of initiating them. In the same way that a puppy play-bows, lowering their front end and raising their hindquarters in the air with expectant eyes, so the fox would run towards me, toss his head back over his shoulders and run away from me, with a similarly gleeful demeanour. If I didn't immediately follow, he would run back towards me and do the same in a beckoning gesture that clearly communicated, 'Come follow me!' And to assist with the fun, something else had happened. My parents' garden was littered with around six colourful children's balls which the fox had gathered from our neighbours' gardens! I would sometimes look out of the window to see him tossing these into the air with his mouth, following them with an exuberant leap off the ground, and then pouncing and batting them when they landed.

On the last evening of September we chased around the fir tree as usual before heavy rain started to fall. I would normally have returned inside for shelter, but the fox had not run for the bushes so I decided to stay outside and flopped down on to the soaking grass instead. He sat down, too, and looked at me as the rain began to belt down in sheets. I talked to him in a gentle voice, as always, and then lay down on my front and extended my open hand towards him. I had never stroked the fox, or ever attempted to. Perhaps in the back of my mind I didn't even know if I should.

It was dark and my hair was now plastered to my head as the rain fell harder and the fox looked at my open palm reaching towards him. He lowered his head and I felt his hard teeth tentatively mouthing my skin. He let go and sat still as I gently stroked his fur with my extended finger tips.

It was the only time I ever stroked him, a moment of trust in the rain, and as I did so I wondered how I would feel if someone was to appear in the garden with aggressive, barking dogs straining at their leash.

Of course, a fox hunt would not suddenly appear in my parents' garden but my instinct would be to protect my companion. To afford him safety and demand to know why this person would want to set dogs on him to take his life. We do not usually have such an intimate relationship with individual foxes or other wild animals, but this one had given me a unique insight into their thinking and feeling nature: an animal who has interests, a personality, who solves problems and derives apparent pleasures from life. To justify extinguishing this rich existence, the person would need an exceptionally good reason for doing so. They would need to be faced by a problem caused by the fox of such severity that no reasonable person would simply be able to ignore it. The problem would not be treatable by any other means, such as by erecting effective fox-proof fencing, and killing the fox would be the only proven solution. Setting the dogs on the fox, knowing that there would be a long chase which would create fear (otherwise the fox would not run away) and be tiring, possibly exhausting, would have to be judged as the most humane achievable method when compared with all other possible methods. An argument that foxes have always been killed this way would not be sufficient. And it should not be primarily to derive entertainment from the chasing and killing, either directly or through associated social gatherings. Entertainment can be created in other ways and the fox's interests are worth more than this. Such logical steps form the basis of the International Consensus Principles for Ethical Wildlife Control, which were agreed in 2017 to help guide approaches to the growing number of human–wildlife conflicts across the world.

These conflicts occur when, for example, the growing human population expands into previously wildlife-rich areas, competing with wild animals for food and space. These could be elephants in Africa and Asia – where elephants who have lost habitat to agricultural expansion may raid crops and be killed for doing so – or smaller mammals, such as rats, mice and possums, who may enter our homes and grain stores, or pose threats to endangered wild species. In each case, fostering a 'culture of coexistence' or practising 'compassionate conservation' does not mean prohibiting killing animals who are involved in these conflicts when this is deemed necessary. Rather that control measures are, deliberately and transparently, ethically justified before deployment and are selected for being those that cause the least possible amount of animal suffering.

When such an ethically rigorous approach is taken, some traditional methods of killing wildlife may be considered to be unjustifiably inhumane, through a combination of the suffering they cause and the widespread availability of more humane alternatives. So-called glue traps, sold cheaply to the public in the UK and elsewhere, give an example. These glue-covered boards, to which animals become stuck, are placed in areas frequented by problem rodents. While they may be effective, they can cause individual animals 'instant and prolonged distress and trauma, followed by dehydration, hunger and sometimes self-mutilation'. Observations have reported some animals' mouths becoming glued shut as a result of trying to chew themselves free, eye damage and raw skin patches where fur was torn away. Given the availability of more humane alternative methods, such as well-constructed and regularly checked spring-powered (or 'break-back') traps, a number of organizations, including OneKind, the RSPCA and the British Veterinary Association, have been lobbying for glue traps to be made illegal. In 2022, the UK government banned the use of glue traps by the general public in England, and the Scottish and Welsh governments have announced their intention to do the same.

To prompt similar review and reform, the International Consensus Principles for Ethical Wildlife Control should be widely promoted and adopted around the world.

The weather became rainier and beech leaves shushed their final whispers. The clouds cleared to reveal a starry October night sky and I heard a thin, high-pitched call penetrating the cold night air. Then another. It was the first time I had heard it this year: another wild call heard every autumn since my childhood. Silk being spun around the stars, the sound produced by a beautiful thrush arriving in our skies from Scandinavia. Migrating redwings.

Redwings never cease to amaze me. First of all, you have to get your ear attuned to them. I have stood outside with people who have been interested in hearing their night-time calls. Clear nights are best and we have stepped out into the cool air to listen.

Thirty seconds later, 'There!' I would exclaim excitedly. 'Did you hear that?'

'Not yet,' they would answer, with an air of disappointment.

Ten seconds later I would rapidly gesture to the sky and spin to look at them with a smile. 'No... not that time,' would come the reply.

I would try to better describe what we were listening out for: a thin, high-pitched 'tseeep', probably higher in pitch than they might expect. And they nod and say, 'OK,' and strain their ears towards the starry heavens.

'There!' I exclaim again.

This time there is a flicker of recognition. They are nodding, 'I think I got that one.'

Nearly a minute passes and then, in unison, our heads spin to face each other, nodding and smiling. 'I heard that one!'

Once you are tuned in, autumn nights are never the same again as those calls pierce the darkness. And it is not a call that you hear as a chance encounter; the skies are filled with them. Taunton Railway Station, the Beatles' Penny Lane, Bushmills in Northern Ireland, over the skies of Formby and above Bristol city centre – all places, urban and rural, that immediately spring to mind as places where I have heard the nocturnal contact calls of journeying redwings. To step out at any place in the British Isles on an autumn night, at any time, and almost be guaranteed to hear one indicates that they are passing overhead in their hundreds of thousands.

The birds are similar to a song thrush, but with a broad creamy stripe above their eye and rusty orange flanks which extend beneath their wings in flight. They are heading for berry-laden hedgerows where they spend the winter, feasting on fruits as red as their feathers and, if disturbed, streaming from the frosty hawthorns while calling, leaving their invisible notes trailing in the cold winter air.

CHAPTER 7

Robins and cows

My first experience with dairy cows was during a placement on a farm of less than 100 cows in the north-west of England. Here I gained my first insight into dairy farming and learned about the nature of cows themselves. I was surprised to find that such large, intimidating animals were in fact gentle and inherently curious about people. Instead of front teeth in their upper jaw, they have a soft dental pad. By drawing tufts of grass into their mouth with their rough tongue and then pressing their lower incisor teeth against this pad to sever the stalks, cattle are able to graze the plants that sustain them. Both the rough tongue and the slobbery pad could be amply appreciated when some of the cows offered me exploratory licks. Occasionally the farmer's elderly mother attended to milk the cows and helped me refine my technique for manual milking while conferring her wisdom. 'A vet should always talk to their animals, whatever kind they're treating,' she would say in a frail voice, 'it gives them confidence. Talk to her, put a hand on her back,' she said, gently demonstrating with a cow in front of her, 'she shouldn't get any surprises.' This advice has served me well, with animals large and small, ever since.

Some years later I was enrolled on the veterinary degree course and heading to my first placement on a dairy farm. Winter had arrived with a vengeance and even in my warm home the air felt cold on my face and feet when I pulled back my blanket on Monday morning; overnight the outside temperature had dropped to −9°C. Shale Farm was inland, across the mosslands, and I drove there beneath early flocks of geese and wildfowl on the coastal road at Southport in hazy morning sunlight. By the time I was nearing the farm the sun was shining brightly in a clear blue sky.

Even wearing gloves, my hands could feel the chilling temperatures as I pulled the grating bar on a metal gate and drew into the muddy farm yard, also frozen hard. There was the silence of desertion that I was now used to and then, after limited wandering shouting 'Hello!', the also now familiar appearance of a ruddy man wearing green wellingtons, blue cargo trousers and a worn green anorak. His face bulged and dipped, with eyes buried in valleys gouged by countless winters.

'He' la,' he offered in a gruff voice, striding towards me. 'Yu cumma 'el us 'av ya? Cumma see a' cows?' I had to concentrate quite hard to understand the strong rural accent.

I shook the farmer's hand.

'Ah ye, well ya can 'el us and we'll show ya wa gus on.' He set off through a narrow passage and I followed him towards a large straw-filled barn, passing smaller stone-walled buildings in various states of disrepair.

A river ran past the farm, flowing through fields that served as feeding grounds for pink-footed geese and wintering whooper swans, both here from Iceland. Within the farm's boundary, there were calves housed in a number of general storage buildings, a milking parlour, a straw-filled barn and an enclosed outdoor exercise and feeding area. The herd of 120 black-

and-white cows could choose whether to be in the barn or in one of the two penned areas outside.

As two different types of chicken give us eggs and meat (laying hens and broiler chickens), so two different types of cattle give us milk and meat – dairy cows and beef cattle. Both are descended from the same wild ancestor, but dairy cows have been selectively bred by humans for high levels of milk production, while beef cattle have been bred for efficiently converting food into well-developed muscle. The cows standing in front of me were Holstein Friesian dairy cows. Many people are familiar with the sight of black-and-white cows in fields as they pass through the countryside in the summer, but some do not realize that in the winter, when grass is not growing, they are housed in a farm building and typically fed conserved grass (grass silage), maize and formulated food pellets. They may be loose-housed in a straw-bedded barn, as at Shale Farm, or, more commonly, housed in a building containing many cubicles – individual compartments that the cows can enter and leave at will. Some farms, like Shale Farm, also provide an outside area for the cows; others do not.

To produce milk, a cow must first give birth to a calf. Dairy cows will normally have their first calf at approximately two years of age, following a nine-month pregnancy. Her calf is usually taken away from her soon after birth and, instead of suckling a calf, her teats are sucked by a milking machine in the parlour, two to three times daily. The cows I was looking at had been milked at 6am and would be milked again at 4pm. The cow will then produce milk for an average of ten months. To keep milking efficiently, she must give birth to another calf. So around three months after giving birth, while still being milked daily, she is inseminated again (usually by artificial insemination) and nine months later she will have her second calf. She is therefore giving milk daily while a calf is also developing in her womb. Milking is typically stopped at around 305 days, when she is then separated from the milking herd and housed with other dry (pregnant) cows for the remaining two months until her next calf is born.

There were four buildings on the farm designated as calf housing, which each looked like they could do with some structural attention. The farmer told me that shortly before my arrival a young calf had succumbed to pneumonia, so a rickety blower fan, trussed up in a corner, whirred noisily in an attempt to improve ventilation.

Calves are, in some ways, an unfortunate by-product of milk production. They are necessary for the cow to produce milk, and female calves can be reared to replace cows in the herd who die or are culled. But what about male calves? If the cow has been mated by a dairy breed, the male calf is of little use for meat and, being male, no use for milking. There are three principal options for a male dairy calf.

The first is to shoot him at birth. The young calf has no economic value and farmers are unable to feed and house animals out of the kindness of their heart. Shooting should result in an instant, painless death, but it seems like a sad waste of life after nine months in the womb, at odds with the principle of sustainable animal agriculture and demoralizing for many farmers. Being shot at birth is currently the fate of an estimated 95,000 male dairy calves (approximately 19 per cent) per year in the UK.

A second option is selling the calf to be exported from the UK to continental Europe, to be raised for veal. Veal is the meat from a calf, but unlike beef it is pale and sold as a delicacy. There is not currently a large market for veal in the UK, but it is popular in countries such as France, the Netherlands and Italy. The journey from the UK to countries such as these is stressful for the calves, but the way they are then housed until they reach slaughter weight is also of concern. Until 2007 in the European Union (and banned in the UK since 1990, but still permissible in many states in the US) veal calves could be housed in so-called veal crates. These are small crates with a slatted or concrete floor and no bedding, in which calves are housed individually. Having been removed from their farm of birth, the calves spend the rest of their time in this crate, unable to turn around, groom themselves, sleep in a normal position or even stand up or lie down without difficulty. They are kept in near darkness and fed a liquid milk diet, rather than being introduced to solid foods. This prevents their digestive system from developing normally, but by restricting their intake of iron their meat stays 'white', as some consumers demand. The low iron levels cause the calves to become clinically anaemic and abnormal repetitive behaviours are seen, linked to the frustration of highly motivated behaviour, including repeatedly rolling their tongues, licking their crate or sucking on their neighbour. The calves exist like this until they are slaughtered at about four months of age.

Although EU law now prohibits veal crates and requires that calves must be kept in groups (unless they are under eight weeks of age, in which case they must be able to turn round and be able to see, hear and touch other calves), they may, after two weeks old, be kept in barren pens without bedding. In the UK on the other hand, veal calves must have sufficient iron in their diet to prevent anaemia, sufficient fibre after 14 days of age to allow their digestive system to develop, space to turn around and be provided with bedding. So this second option for male dairy calves permits them to be exported hundreds of miles to be raised in conditions which would be illegal had they remained in the UK. This trade has declined significantly in recent years.

The third option is for the calves to be raised for veal in the UK. Here they would be provided with, at least, the living conditions laid out in UK legislation, and British veal reared under the RSPCA Assured scheme is also available. The idea of high-welfare veal seems hard to contemplate, given that veal has been synonymous with the deprivations endured in the veal crate for many years, but it is a fact that calves raised in groups with companionship, bedding and a nutritionally adequate diet could have a good life rather than being shot at birth. Because they are allowed to move around and eat a more normal diet, higher-welfare veal is pink rather than white (sometimes called 'rose veal'). Veterinary bodies and animal welfare charities alike are promoting the benefits of higher-welfare British rose veal to support good lives, and prevent wasteful deaths, for male dairy calves.

A further possibility for alleviating the problem of unwanted male dairy calves is to utilize breeding technology to prevent them from being born in the first place. Sexed semen is increasingly being used to increase the chances that female calves will be born instead of males. The practice has become popular in the UK, with sales of sexed semen doubling in the two years to 2021, to 63.5 per cent of all dairy semen sales, and promotion of the technique in the industry-led GB Dairy Calf Strategy.

'Ve's here, la!'

I spun round to find the farmer's stocky frame blocking out the winter sun.

'Yu wanna com an' 'el us wida calves?'

'Yes, OK,' I replied enthusiastically. I set off following him back down through the passageway and into one of the outbuildings where the three-week-old calves had been gathered into individual metal pens. A vet from a local farm animal practice was stooped, arranging objects in a plastic bucket, and he gave me a welcoming smile as he stood up. 'Hi, I'm Peter,' he said, extending his hand. 'How are you getting on?'

'Yeah, not too bad thanks, I've not been here very long.' A cold wind gusted through the open-fronted building.

'We're just going to disbud a few of these calves, have you done it before?'

'No,' I replied.

'Well if you just want to stand to the side there, you can give me a hand holding them and I'll show you how it's done.'

I stepped closer to the nearest pen and stood to the side of the young calf's head which was poking through. Her pink tongue licked at Peter as he continued to busy himself in the bucket just in front of her, leaving dark saliva patches on his waterproof parlour top. Peter stood up again, holding a needle and syringe.

'OK. If you can see where my finger is, there's a groove running behind the eye up towards where the horn will grow. That's where the nerve runs, so we need to inject local anaesthetic in the groove, about an inch behind the eye, see?'

He held the calf's head firmly against his thigh as he inserted the needle into the skin behind her eye and angled it in different directions as he depressed the plunger. 'Fanning it about makes sure we get good penetration around the nerve,' he said. 'Just have to wait a few minutes now.'

Local anaesthetic needs time to diffuse through the tissues to infiltrate the nerves it will affect. The cornual nerve provides sensation to the skin of the horn region, so by blocking it with a local anaesthetic the calf is unable to feel what happens next. As the minutes passed, Peter fired up a butane gas canister and inserted a metal iron into it until it was glowing red. The iron had a cylindrical metal end, like an apple corer, and Peter twisted it around slowly in the roaring flame.

Then Robert, the farmer, stepped into the pen behind the calf and carefully pulled the calf's head to one side with one hand, while lowering her ear, to move it out of the way. Peter pricked the calf's skin with a needle to ensure there was no twitching and, satisfied that she was sensation-free, applied the hot iron to the calf's head. It hissed and momentarily surrounded us with the choking acrid smoke of burning hair and tissue. More twisting, this time with the iron firmly pressed against her head, gouging the corer left and right, up and down, then in less than ten seconds it was withdrawn with a flick of the wrist, removing a plug of skin and leaving behind a ring of expertly burned flesh. Peter repeated the process for the opposite side and moved on to the other animals. I helped to restrain a few and within an hour the job of disbudding the small group of calves was complete.

I walked back to the cow yard and stood watching the cows again. From a post opposite, a robin's pensive song drifted in wispy columns of condensation from the bird's opening and closing beak. It seemed as though routinely mutilating animals was the only way of being able to farm them. What was the justification for what I had just seen?

The reasons given for keeping cows without horns are primarily concerned with human and animal safety. A cow without horns is less likely to injure stockpeople and other animals, and horns are a principal cause of carcass wastage due to bruising, which carries an economic cost. Hornless cows also require less space at feeding troughs.

Although some people would object to removing a calf's horns like this because they are an integral part of the animal and the calf should be allowed to keep them, others would be more concerned about the pain and suffering caused by the procedure. What is known about that?

A distinction is made between disbudding and dehorning. Disbudding was the procedure that Peter had just performed with the hot iron and involves removing the horn-producing cells before a horn has developed. The early developing horn is called a horn bud and disbudding involves removing it before it attaches to the bone beneath. This attachment occurs at around two months of age. If the resulting horn is then removed this is called dehorning. Best practice is to disbud so that dehorning, which is more invasive, does not become necessary. Most of a cow's horn is not dead or inert, as some people think, but living and supplied with sensory nerves and blood vessels.

There are different methods for removing horns and horn buds, and most have been scientifically assessed for the pain they are likely to cause. One important physiological measure is the extent to which the animal produces the hormone cortisol following the procedure. Cortisol is produced in response to physical or psychological challenges.

When a hot disbudding iron is applied to a calf's head, without local anaesthetic having first been administered, there is a rush of cortisol production. Blood levels gradually decrease and return to normal within two hours. Measurements of heart rate, which indicate arousal of the sympatho-adrenal system – which also responds to stressful challenges – reveal that the heart rate stays higher than in control calves (ones who have been restrained in the same way and had their horn buds firmly handled, but not burned) for three and a half hours, beyond the initial cortisol spike. This suggests that hot-iron disbudding without anaesthetic is acutely painful and the pain may last for at least three hours. A calf's behaviour supports this conclusion, with initial application of the iron, without local anaesthetic, causing 'rearing, falling down, pushing and head jerking' and calves continuing to shake their heads in the two hours following the procedure.

Further research indicates that calves find the overall procedure aversive and learn to avoid locations where it has been performed. In three connected test pens – one where calves were disbudded with local anaesthetic, one where they underwent a 'mock' procedure and a neutral pen where nothing happened – calves chose to spend less time in either of the treatment pens compared to the neutral pen. When comparing only the two treatment pens, the calves spent less time in the disbudding pen and were less likely to lie down there. The researchers conclude that, 'Even with the use of a local anaesthetic, hot-iron disbudding is [...] aversive for calves, indicating the need to refine or avoid the procedure.'

I would join those who say it seems patently obvious that burning a calf's head with a red-hot iron is painful; you don't need science to prove *that*! But when pitted against others who argue the opposite, or dispute the degree of pain caused, the science becomes invaluable in informing guidelines and regulations by which people must abide for as long as the mutilation is deemed unavoidable.

In the UK a person does not have to be a vet to perform disbudding, but using local anaesthesia to numb the area first, as I had seen, is a legal requirement. For those wishing to lobby for changes in countries where this is not the case, the scientific evidence needs to be communicated to inform fact-based arguments.

After a few months, cattle have recognisable horns, and during later parts of my training, on different farms, I have been required to remove these (to perform dehorning) using guillotine shears or embryotomy wire. The first implement is a pair of heavy-duty metal shears similar to those used to lop tree branches. The second is like a large cheese wire, moved vigorously backward and forward to slice through the horn. In the studies already mentioned, dehorning, if performed without local anaesthetic, causes the greatest cortisol response of all methods, lasting seven to nine hours. This is due to the initial physical trauma of the procedure and then the uncontrolled inflammation that follows. The cattle (as reported in the scientific literature) shake their head and tail in the hours following dehorning, flick their ears and rub themselves against their pen.

In the UK, local anaesthetic must be used during the dehorning procedure. Certainly, when used with both hot-iron disbudding and amputation dehorning, local anaesthesia reduces both the cortisol response and the calf's attempts to struggle or escape, by numbing sensation. But the problem with a local anaesthetic is that after some hours it wears off. The way to tackle the ongoing pain is to additionally administer a non-steroidal anti-inflammatory drug (NSAID, similar to aspirin used by people).

Awareness of pain in cattle is growing, including within the veterinary profession. Research suggests that the perception of, and willingness to treat, pain by UK cattle practitioners has increased in the last decade. The British Veterinary Association (BVA), together with the British Cattle Veterinary Association (BCVA), now recommend the use of NSAIDs in addition to local anaesthesia when conducting disbudding and castration in calves, as does the American Association of Bovine Practitioners, since 2019. All three organizations also recommend increasingly breeding from naturally 'polled' (hornless) animals, so that calves aren't born with horns. In 2019, using local anaesthetic when disbudding and dehorning cattle became a legal requirement in New Zealand. Meanwhile, the BVA and BCVA are calling for UK legislation to go further, advocating that current legislation – requiring local anaesthetic but not an NSAID – does not reflect a level of appropriate analgesia and 'fails to reflect changes in scientific understanding, pharmaceutical developments and societal opinions'. Further global societal pressure will increase the likelihood of these recommendations being realized sooner rather than later.

One morning a spreading pool of crimson blood developed beneath the elevated back foot of a cow immobilized in a metal cattle crush. She had been confined by Robert, who was treating her for a foot complaint: digital dermatitis. He ushered me over to look at the underside of her hoof, which was lifted from the ground and tied with fraying rope. The soft tissues between her claws and heel were raw and bleeding, and he told me that he would need to clean the affected area before he could apply a therapeutic antibiotic spray. The cow tried to kick and clatter within the crush as the jet from a hose flushed her diseased tissues.

She wasn't alone in her affliction. Several other cows could be seen lifting a back leg and flicking their foot, or walking gingerly to avoid placing their tender feet on the ground. Digital dermatitis is one of the most common causes of lameness in UK dairy cattle and I was witnessing well-recognized behavioural signs of the substantial pain it can cause. Nationwide, lameness – described as one of the most pressing issues in the dairy industry – affects approximately a third of UK dairy cows, despite committed industry effort and focus, equivalent to around three-quarters of a million dairy cows in the UK being lame at any one time.

Other cows in the herd were afflicted with different ailments. Several had pieces of coloured tape wrapped around their tail, indicating that their milk was to be discarded. These cows were being treated with antibiotics for mastitis – inflammation of the udders, which can also be very painful – so their milk could not enter the food chain until the treatment course had ended. Robert was also having difficulty getting some of his cows to fall pregnant.

Like all farmers, Robert was doing his very best to tend to his cows and provide them with the best care he could, but he was at the mercy of a troubled industry. At lunchtime on my final day, he invited me into his farmhouse kitchen, adorned with hanging pots, pans and horse brasses, and sat me down at a large oak table. He began expressing the understandable frustration that I had become accustomed to at the end of my various farm placements.

Like most of the farmed species I had already encountered, in recent decades dairy cattle have been selectively bred for ever-increasing productivity. In 1980, a dairy cow would have produced around 4,000 litres (7,000 pints) of milk in a year; she now produces over 8,000 litres (14,000 pints). The European Food Safety Authority's Animal Health and Welfare Panel concluded that, 'Long-term genetic selection for high milk yield is the major factor causing poor welfare, in particular health problems, in dairy cows.' As for other species, many years focussing on a single production trait has inadvertently selected for an increased susceptibility to health and welfare problems, including, in dairy cows, conditions such as lameness, mastitis and reproductive disorders. In recognition of this, breeding goals have now widened to include health and welfare, but sustained progress relies on milk being properly valued.

Dramatic increases in productivity have not been matched by increases in profitability. As a result, the UK has lost more than half of its dairy farmers since the mid-1990s. The economic reasons for this are complex, but include the price paid by milk buyers and processors. Again, we must highlight the role of citizens (both at the level of individual shoppers and that of supermarkets and other retailers), and several veterinary commentators have noted that, as a society, we are currently happy to pay significantly more for bottled water than we are for milk. The injustice here, however, is that the price premium flowing towards bottled water cannot be harnessed to improve the lives of the male dairy calves, pay for the adequate pain relief needed for disbudding and dehorning – or fund work on expanding alternative approaches – and tackle the diseases, and their underlying causes, linked to the high productive output of the gentle dairy cow.

Many readers will be familiar with proposals put forward to respond to this economic crisis in dairy farming. In February 2010, a planning application was submitted to develop the largest dairy farm in Europe in Lincolnshire, UK. Housing 8,100 cows, it was to be a so-called super- or mega-dairy, achieving improved viability through economies of scale.

The super-dairy would be purpose-built and boast some of the most modern facilities for housing and milking dairy cattle. As Professors Jon Huxley and Martin Green wrote in the *Veterinary Record*, 'New purpose-built units of any size often have significant advantages over older units which have grown organically over many decades.' This would not be a place of crumbling brickwork like Shale Farm and many others. In addition, the super-dairy would have its own dedicated cattle vets, tasked, alongside competent and compassionate stockpeople, with keeping disease levels as low as possible. But would this lead to an improved quality of life for the cows?

What concerned many about the super-dairy proposal was that the cattle were to be kept in very large numbers – too many, they felt, to be adequately cared for as individuals – and they were to be permanently housed in buildings. Unlike the present situation, where many cows are housed indoors during the winter then turned out to pasture in the spring, thousands of cows in a super-dairy would spend their entire life indoors, with exercise areas at best, rather than grassy fields upon which to range.

Professors Jon Huxley and Martin Green were keen to stress that they did not wish to advocate this, or any other particular type of farm, but it did seem that optimum facilities and well-resourced healthcare should benefit cows. But some issues remained. If the cows being housed and cared for were the same high-yielding breeds whose productivity has come at the expense of their health, then this genetic impact on quality of life would be the same however the cows were housed. Continued genetic selection for health alongside milk yield would be needed to tackle this.

A shift in breeding emphasis was promising, but the issue of permanent housing remained. Could cows in super-dairies have good wellbeing? In an advisory letter to the UK government Minister of State for Agriculture and Food in August 2010, the government's advisory Farm Animal Welfare Council (now Animal Welfare Committee) identified two key issues that would influence this.

The first was large group size. This, they felt, should not be incompatible with satisfactory standards of animal welfare, so long as the total herd is divided into smaller manageable groups and 'stockmanship is of the highest standard'.

The second issue was all-year-round housing. This, they said, posed a risk to the fourth of the Five Freedoms – the ability to express normal behaviour – but research to establish how this impacts on welfare in permanently housed cows had not been undertaken. They speculated that a 'satisfactory' standard of welfare could be achieved, but not the Committee's proposed higher standard of a 'good life'.

Research has subsequently shown that dairy cows demonstrate a strong motivation to access pasture and show indicators of improved emotional wellbeing when they are able to do so. Recall the consumer demand approach to assessing strength of motivation, from Chapter 2, where animals work increasingly hard to access resources they value. In 2017, researchers in Canada found, using this methodology, that the motivation of cattle to push through weighted gates to access pasture was as high as their motivation to access fresh food after milking. Immediately after milking is the time when cattle are most motivated to eat. When cows were given the opportunity at this time to push through ever-heavier gates to access pasture, they did so despite fresh food being freely available to them inside their barn. This indicated that their motivation was to access pasture per se and engage in behaviours such as grazing, rather than simply because they were hungry.

Researchers from Queen's University Belfast used another fascinating approach, called cognitive bias – which we look at in the next chapter – to see if continuously housed dairy cows were more or less pessimistic than those given pasture access. Those in the continuously housed group responded in ways indicative of reduced psychological wellbeing. Dr Andrew Crump commented, 'We hope that our research encourages farmers, retailers, government and consumers that pasture access is important for cow welfare, and should be protected.'

Several studies have also shown that reduced access to pasture is a risk factor for lameness, with the Federation of Veterinarians of Europe advocating the benefits of well-managed pasture access and well-managed straw yards as an important aspect of lameness prevention.

Ninety-five per cent of the British public believe pasture access benefits dairy cows and over 80 per cent of the public in Germany, the United States, Canada and Brazil believe the same, with implications for the ethical sustainability of dairy farming.

The studies of cow motivation and wellbeing suggest this may be a sound view, so long as, of course, pasture is well managed and the cows are provided with adequate shelter. However, it is a fact that currently, worldwide, most milk now comes from dairy cows who are housed exclusively indoors. Less than 5 per cent of the 10 million lactating cows in the United States, for example, have access to pasture. Some countries, though, have taken a different view, such as Sweden, where full-time housing is banned. In the UK, a decade after the Lincolnshire proposal, around 95 per cent of UK dairy cows are still – at the moment – going out to pasture at some point during the year.

In February 2011, plans for the Lincolnshire super-dairy were withdrawn. This was not due to objections over animal welfare, but because the developers had failed to persuade the Environment Agency that there would not be an unacceptable risk of pollution to groundwater. The local district council also had concerns about odour, noise and threats to wildlife.

What might the future of dairy farming hold? As sustainability has risen up the political agenda, there is a growing focus on so-called regenerative agriculture, utilizing farming methods that help combat the climate emergency, prevent further biodiversity loss, protect human health and give all farm animals a good quality of life. If we feel that cows should be able to enjoy the clement months out in fields, producing milk from grass for us to drink, then why should this not be? If we value the biodiversity – the birds and insects – that live in fields grazed by cattle, then their losses should also be carefully considered. Some propose that emissions of greenhouse gases from cattle can be better managed if the cows are housed, but the potential for grazed pasture to absorb and lock in environmental carbon should not be neglected. To help reduce the problem of unwanted male dairy calves, a growing proportion of dual-purpose dairy cattle are being bred: animals who still produce good volumes of milk, but also develop muscle that is suitable for good-quality beef. Another approach is to mate dairy cows with bulls of a beef breed, so that the male calves can be reared for beef. In these cases, milk production is less than that obtained from the present high-yielding animals, but income can be derived from the sale of the calves and more of the milk can be produced from the farm's own grass rather than relying so heavily on bought-in foods that have their own environmental footprint.

The future, incorporating all of these concerns, is intimately linked to economics. As well as the need for governments to allocate agricultural subsidies to support sustainability goals, including animal welfare and biodiversity alongside productivity, we, as citizens and consumers, also have a key role to play. We can use on-packet logos to guide our purchases. RSPCA Assured and Soil Association labels in the UK, and the Global Animal Partnership five-step animal welfare rating programme in the US, for example, include commitments on disbudding, lameness prevention and pasture access during the grazing season. And we can choose to shop in stores that have been recognized for prioritizing animal welfare in their supply chains; many are ranked in the free-to-download Business Benchmark on Farm Animal Welfare Report. Some UK supermarkets, for example, are auditing and reducing lameness levels, require the use of NSAIDs for disbudding and prohibit the killing of unwanted male calves at birth. These are practical ways for us to express that the quality of life of dairy cows and the quality of their living environment should be financially supported to the same extent that we support the industry that, each year, sells us millions of litres of bottled water.

CHAPTER 8

Starlings and slaughter

I was looking forward to spending Christmas at home with my family, but had one last placement to do: the abattoir. I had a few free days first and as noon slipped into early afternoon I was drawn to a daily wild spectacle at the Silver Jubilee Bridge near Liverpool.

I look out on to the river below and across towards the bridge sweeping up towards the sky and down again towards the industrial town of Runcorn. Often likened to the Sydney Harbour Bridge, it forms a distinctive arch of latticed steel forming a prominent local landmark, beneath which a never-ending flow of traffic crosses elegant viaducts and a roadway suspended by wire ropes that descend like harp strings.

In the clear winter sky, hundreds of gulls fly purposefully on slow, arched wings towards the estuary upriver. They form an uninterrupted escalator of birds, quietly moving towards the safety of their roost, past the twinkling lights of the nearby chemical factories. I keep my gloved hands in my pockets as I watch them passing overhead, for an hour or more.

Their presence slows the pace, together with the sentry-like heron on the riverbank. The sky begins to turn pastel orange and the background rumble of lorries crossing the bridge is woven into a growing urban peace.

A small group of around 50 arrowhead-like birds fly in an evenly spaced cluster above me and tilt in unison towards the northern side of the bridge, where they alight. They stay there for a couple of minutes, then lift again, making a few synchronized flaps of their wings before gliding like dark paper aeroplanes out over the river in a compact group. They bank, still in perfect synchrony, and twist back towards the bridge. Across the river, above Runcorn, I can see another dark group of birds doing the same. There are more in this group; I guess a couple of hundred. Their motion is identical, flying as a close-knit flock. The gulls keep coming, passing from east to west.

Each paper aeroplane is a starling: a bird of jerky walking, noisy chattering and with a domineering reputation at bird tables. Some people dislike them, preferring that smaller, shyer birds get some of the food that the starlings devour as a noisy mob. In the sunset skies above the bridge the starlings are silent, their characterful ebullience replaced by a unified focus of mind and movement.

Several hundred-strong groups are now spinning like tops in the sky either side of the bridge, toing and froing in coordinated flocks, away and towards the bridge. Then, above the rooftops of Runcorn directly ahead, a small patch of the cold pale sky becomes pixelated. I focus my attention on it and strain my eyes. The graininess develops into a faint wisp of smoke that drifts above the town, growing at its leading edge as it draws closer towards the bridge, tapering away to a distant, imagined, point. To my right, the sun has begun to dip low behind the bridge, sending a warm orange glow through the viaduct's stone arches.

A thousands-strong flock of starlings is now swirling mesmerically above the sweeping arch of the bridge which, like a giant satellite receiver, has become a focal point for flocking starlings from across the globe. A number of the birds will be residents, staying in the UK to breed in the spring, but many more are winter migrants from Russia and Scandinavia who have fled the bitter temperatures of their homelands.

This super-flock has assimilated all of the foregoing flocks and moves like a dark monolith, occasionally obscuring the reddening clouds. The flock's form is soft with smooth, rounded edges. I could be on a rocky peninsula watching rolling waves gather and crash. The starling flock sweeps skyward, allowing currents of birds to move into the space created beneath, then narrows through invisible gaps and eddies. Flowing in this way, the mass of starlings moves away from the bridge, towards me, darkening the sky above the Mersey. It reaches an undefined point and then contorts, flicking out a long tail of birds that whips in slow motion through the gap between the opposing riverbanks. The ceiling of birds is pulled in one direction, then another, but the direction of movement is always back towards the bridge. The entire flock descends upon the upper arch, creating a long line of iron filings across a giant magnet.

I have visited enough times to know that the starlings will not roost on the arch itself, but in the so-called box girders supporting the road beneath. The steel girders are hollow and the hundreds-of-thousands-strong flock will spend the night huddled inside them. The flock lifts as one again and draws out across the river, the birds moving in a slowly morphing mass. The scene is all-consuming and incomprehensible.

We cannot know how it feels to be one of the starlings, but their collective behaviour gives an indication of the individual's likely psyche.

The bridge affords great benefits, including shelter and protection from predators while they sleep, but to gather in such numbers every evening carries its own risk. Their nightly arrival becomes predictable for sparrowhawks and peregrine falcons who learn to strike the swirling flocks before the starlings reach the protection of the steel girders. The starlings seem to recognize this risk, forming larger and more compact flocks when predators are present and the birds give the impression that none wants to be the first to land.

Each bird has a reaction time of under 100 milliseconds, and shapes begin to form as the murmuration balls and hurries. A kidney passes from right to left. Then a sprawling red blood cell, oxygenating the peach sky. A pair of lungs, heaving and sighing, expanding and contracting. The arch of the bridge repeats again and again as the birds dip and swoop over its invisible reflections. The flock stretches out, billowing and rippling like the flapping bed sheets in the nearby backyards, and as it draws out above my tilted head, extending to every horizon, I am lulled by the shushing of thousands of intermittently flapping and gliding wings. To hear the air beneath a creature's beating wings, whether bird, bat or butterfly, is to sense ultimate peace and solitude.

The sun has reached the river. Floodlights illuminate the bridge, broadcasting its structural prowess. Some of the birds are going to have to land soon; they know it and their wheeling and gyrating becomes more urgent. Now the magnet is a conductor's baton, flinging and swiping through the filings, which trail without choice. Nature's patterns crescendo, ending as quickly as they began, and the bridge extracts the smoke from the sky, giving refuge to thousands of huddling starlings.

Inevitably, humans have sought to elucidate the meaning of the starlings' behaviour and complex vocalizations at their roost. Infrared and thermal-imaging cameras reveal that, through jostling and posturing, dominant adults occupy the warmest locations in the roost, while younger birds must huddle together in the more exposed extremities. In addition to conserving body heat, the roosting starlings, who could travel around 30 miles to and from their feeding areas each day, appear to exchange information on the best feeding locations.

Such findings serve to remind us that, despite their highly coordinated arrivals and departures, the dense flocks comprise thousands, sometimes millions of animals, each an individual in their own right. Uniformly black from a distance, starlings up close are among the most beautiful of British birds. Their metallic plumage shimmers green and violet, with hundreds of yellowish-white arrows streaming across their head and body.

Some starlings are captured from the wild and transferred to laboratory aviaries for biological research. They are among the most popular bird species used for this purpose, in areas such as avian infectious diseases, foraging behaviour, the neurobiology of song production and the environmental control of breeding and moulting. Given their popularity in experimental research, they have also, in recent years, become the subject of animal welfare science research, which has sought to establish how captivity may impact upon their wellbeing.

One of the outcomes of this research has been to develop a fascinating scientific approach to understanding animal emotions. Previous chapters have highlighted the value of indicators such as stereotypical behaviour, stress hormone levels and self-medication. Another interesting approach to understanding an animal's feelings, explored in starling welfare research, assesses their degree of optimism.

This scientific approach builds on the fact that people experiencing anxiety and depression typically view circumstances more pessimistically than people not experiencing these feelings. When given choices that ambiguously predict whether an outcome is likely to be positive or negative, people experiencing depression are more likely to predict a negative outcome; they are more likely to have a glass-half-empty perspective on the world. This is described as a cognitive bias and researchers at Newcastle University examined whether a similar bias occurred in captive starlings, and whether it was likely to be indicative of negative feelings, such as anxiety or depression.

The experimental starlings were first trained that a light appearing in their test cage would remain illuminated for either two or ten seconds. They were given two buttons to peck – one red and one green. If the light stayed on for two seconds they were taught to press the red button and receive a tasty food pellet straight away, and if it stayed on for ten seconds they would press the green button and get their food reward a few seconds later. If they got it wrong there was a long delay before they could try again. Unsurprisingly, the birds preferred to receive the food pellet as soon as possible, and this was used to investigate their degree of optimism.

Once the birds had learned their task, the second stage of the experiment manipulated the length of time that the light remained illuminated, between two and ten seconds. Three seconds of illumination is similar to two, so, predictably, the starlings pecked the red button, as though the answer was two. But what about six seconds? Would they choose the red or the green? Remember, with the promise of a food treat they were keen to get it right.

The experimental technique became interesting from an animal welfare perspective because the researchers divided their starlings between two different housing types. One half of the group were housed in standard cages, with a simple dowel perch and newspaper on the floor. The other half were housed in enriched cages, which were larger, had perches made from natural branches of differing thicknesses, had continuous access to a water bath and bark chippings on the floor. Whereas the first group had mealworms to eat provided in a bowl, the mealworms in the enriched environment were scattered through the bark chippings so that the starlings could forage more naturally.

The researchers found that when the light task became ambiguous, the birds housed in the standard cages were more likely to anticipate that the reward was going to be delayed; they were more pessimistic.

Next, the researchers investigated abnormal repetitive behaviour, a well-utilized indicator of poor welfare discussed in Chapter 2. Some captive starlings exhibited repetitive somersaulting in their cages. To better understand whether this abnormal behaviour was likely to be associated with emotions akin to depression or anxiety, the Newcastle team devised another cognitive bias experiment. In this case, the somersaulting birds were those who responded more pessimistically to ambiguous shades of grey, when black was associated with a large food reward and white with a reward that was more meagre.

As always, these experiments cannot give us definitive proof of how these animals are feeling. But they raise the important possibility, relevant to debates about the morality of caging birds, that barren cages result in negative mental states and those birds who develop apparently purposeless repetitive behaviour are experiencing feelings which we would find unpleasant.

Colourful Christmas lights brought necklaces of cheer to gardens and homes as I drove through quiet streets on my first morning's drive to the abattoir. Bare trees, like feathery gills, stood motionless beneath blanched skies, dotted with old nests.

Despite rising early, by the time I arrived at the abattoir at 8:30am the day's cattle had all been slaughtered. Luis, the veterinary surgeon with responsibility for enforcing animal welfare and public health legislation at the plant was unfazed. 'Don't worry, there'll be more tomorrow!' he said enthusiastically. He was keen to explain his official duties to me and thumbed through several bulging files of theory and legislation as he cheerfully confronted me with strings of facts and figures before suggesting we leave his small office and take a tour of the sprawling site.

Most people are concerned that the lives of animals who feed us should be good lives; that although these animals are born to die, they should be treated considerately and humanely while they are alive. This spreading animal welfare-based philosophy, reflective of our own moral progress, should logically extend to the animals' lives in their entirety. As well as a good life, it follows that animals whom we kill for food should also have a humane death.

The UK currently slaughters in the order of 2.8 million cattle, 11 million pigs, 14.5 million sheep and lambs and 1 billion birds for human consumption every year. For the welfare of these animals to be acceptable up until the point of their death, they must be transported, unloaded, handled, moved and killed carefully and compassionately. For this to be possible for so many animals, well-run and monitored systems must be in place at the abattoir, and part of Luis' job was to ensure that this was the case.

We walked across in wellington boots to an outdoor receiving pen where a large lorry was lowering its tailgate to the ground. It was the type of lorry that is often seen on motorways, with slatted sides that give glimpses of curly fleeces or skyward-pointing nostrils. Once gates and rails had been secured, the ramp reverberated with the clatter of thousands of hoofs as a torrent of sheep jostled and bucked to exit into the open pen beneath. Luis watched closely to check none were showing signs of lameness or injury.

The sheep were guided into smaller pens in an area known as the lairage, which served as a waiting area while those ahead of them began to enter the abattoir itself. We walked through the lairage, to the point where the first sheep were being ushered into high-sided races (passageways) and watched as they moved in a steady stream towards the building before disappearing from sight. To ensure this short journey was efficient and stress-free, the races gently curved so that each animal could see just one or two animals ahead and were maintained to ensure no cracks in the sides could admit chinks of light, which could cause the animals to balk.

At this point, Luis indicated that we had reached as far as we could go and I followed him back out onto the yard outside. He explained the importance of strict hygiene procedures inside the abattoir as we crossed the yard and into a small room where a row of white overalls hung from pegs. A few minutes later, all of my work clothes were concealed beneath a set of the overalls, a pair of white wellingtons, a pale hair net and a white hard hat. Then he opened a door and held it for me as I stepped past him and into the alien environment beyond.

We were standing at the edge of an enormous factory, which swallowed us within a din of hissing steam and clunking chains that reverberated around its stainless steel panelling. An unending row of carcasses in various states of disembowelment and butchering snaked jerkily around the metalwork, tended by lines of men in white aprons and hard hats wearing ear defenders. Luis and I began to walk across the factory floor on a designated route among the workers and suspended dead animals, but few of the workers looked up from their varied tasks of cutting, hoisting and inspecting. Despite the disorientating noise and steam, I got the sense that we were walking in the direction of the animals' entrance and as we turned a corner I could see intermittent daylight through an opening ahead, as, one by one, live sheep were conveyed to the waiting machinery and metalwork.

Luis signalled that we should pause, and then explained to me that the next workers we would encounter would be those responsible for stunning and killing the animals. I ascended a small number of steps with him and then looked down on to the race below.

Having entered the building from outside, two panels in contact with the sheep's sides ensured that the animals remained facing forwards. The panels tapered towards the bottom, forming a V-shape, which supported the animals' bodies as their feet were lifted off the ground and a conveyor advanced them forward. The conveyor delivered the animals to the space just below where we were standing, and, being restrained, they were calm and quiet, at least to look at. At this point, the staff member standing in front of us reached for a large pair of metal tongs, like a pair of crossed hockey sticks, and applied them across the sheep's head, in the spaces between the ears and eyes. The tongs delivered an electric current through the sheep's brain that rendered them instantly unconscious before they could register any pain. The current triggered an epileptic fit, causing the sheep to collapse instantly and the animal's back legs to curl up towards their body. The sheep was still completely unconscious and the workers now moved swiftly to attach a metal shackle to one of the sheep's back legs and begin mechanically hoisting the animal up towards an overhead rail, so that they were suspended with their head and forelegs pointing towards the floor. The sheep then began to enter the second stage of stunning and, while still unconscious, began involuntarily kicking their back legs vigorously, causing the metal chains to rattle and bang noisily. Satisfied that the sheep was well secured and still unconscious, one of the workers drew a large knife from its protective sheath and sliced across the sheep's neck causing crimson blood to come gushing from the animal's major vessels. With little time to dwell on what I had seen, the chain in the overhead rail then began moving, the body of the sheep drew away into the steamy gloom and the next live animal arrived at the stunning point below.

The following day, Luis notified me that a consignment of cattle was being slaughtered and we made our way back to the stunning area. The process was similar to the sheep, but the cattle entered the stunning pen individually, on foot, rather than in the V-shaped restrainer. Once in position, this time the slaughterman used a captive bolt stunner rather than electrical tongs. With a cow in the pen, their ears flicking and twitching in response to the noises ahead, the captive bolt gun was rapidly applied to the forehead, causing a steel bolt to burst from the device on contact. This penetrated the skull and continued through into the animal's brain, before recoiling back into the gun. Such a mechanism, as for electrical stunning, causes instant loss of consciousness without pain, and the huge animals instantly crumpled to the pen floor. Next, the side of the pen opened and the unconscious animal rolled out, to be met by the workers waiting to shackle a hind leg and hoist the great beast onto the overhead rail. The cattle then had their major blood vessels severed with a large knife, causing another deluge of blood to come gushing down onto the floor of the bleeding area.

Beyond the stunning and bleeding areas, the freshly dead animals were carried along by the clunking cogs and chains through a production line of sequential processes, which Luis took me to see. First the animals' hides were removed by human cutting and mechanical pulling, then the head was removed, the animal sawn in half with a large rotating saw and their warm organs removed and inspected for signs of disease. Beyond the noisy atmosphere of pistons and hoists, the carcass then entered a chiller for controlled chilling, after which it was deboned, sliced and vacuum packed into the packages we are familiar with on shop shelves.

Luis had picked up on my interest in the slaughter process and, wishing to assist as much as he could, had kindly arranged for me to accompany a meat hygiene inspector to a local poultry abattoir that evening, as Luis' abattoir killed only sheep and cattle. Mine was not a morbid fascination, but a desire to know as much as possible about the experiences of animals at the time of their deaths as well as during their lives.

The poultry abattoir was closer to the centre of town and we arrived at 7pm for slaughtering that would run through the night. The coloured plastic crates that had transported the broiler chickens on lorries from their farms were being off-loaded by forklift trucks when I arrived. Intermittently illuminated by rotating orange warning lights were tens of thousands of white chickens looking out from within the stacks of crates.

When we entered the abattoir from the lairage area, we were confronted by another noisy factory production line and the spectacle of, this time, thousands of suspended chicken bodies snaking through the various stages of processing. I had already forgotten just how many chickens we farm and kill, and still had a sense of incredulity at the never-ending stream of birds passing through this single slaughterhouse. At the beginning of the line, the waiting birds were being pulled from their plastic crates and both their feet slotted into suspended fixtures, so that the birds were hanging upside down. Unlike the cattle and sheep, this happened before stunning, while they were still fully conscious; from here, the moving shackle line carried them towards a water-filled bath.

The bath contained a submerged electrode and as the shackle line moved along above it, the birds' heads dipped into the electrified water, causing an electric current to pass from their submersed heads to the leg shackles. This instantly stunned the brain, resulting in the emergence of unconscious birds the other side, who passed through a mechanical cutter to sever the major blood vessels in their neck. By the time I returned home at 10pm, around 12,000 chickens had been slaughtered since my arrival.

The following day, Luis had once again arranged for me to gain extra insight by sending me to a local pig abattoir. Unlike his place of work, which was large and modern, processing meat for major retailers, the pig slaughterhouse was for a very local market and located behind a butcher's shop in a nearby town. The same requirements had to be met for unloading and handling, and there were pens in the shop's backyard to serve as a lairage, but overall the facilities were more cluttered and dilapidated. Groups of three to four pigs at a time were ushered into a small stunning pen, in which the slaughterman also stood. He used electric tongs for stunning, the same as those used for the sheep at the red meat abattoir, but there were no restraining devices and, instead, he had to position himself over the freely movable pigs before carefully and decisively applying the electrified tongs. This caused the pig to become rigid and fall over, followed by the now-familiar involuntary kicking as the animal was hoisted by their back leg and had their major vessels cut. As I watched animals bleeding out at each of the abattoirs, I experienced a strange sense of relief at the thought that any suffering they had been experiencing was now rushing away.

Slaughter in the United Kingdom is carefully regulated by legislation that aims to prevent personnel involved in the entire slaughter process from causing animals any 'avoidable pain, distress or suffering'. Regardless of how unethical some feel slaughter is or how queasy it may make some people feel, the legislation also requires that animals are competently stunned using methods like those I had witnessed, in order that they do not experience any pain or suffering at the moment their necks are cut.

In a controversial exemption, the legislation permits slaughter without prior stunning if this is undertaken for religious purposes. Within both Judaism and Islam, religious rules determine which animal species may be eaten and how they must be killed. Jewish people cannot eat certain animals, such as pigs or camels, while Muslim people cannot eat certain animals including pigs or any animal which is carnivorous. Meat which has been produced in accordance with Jewish religious rules is termed kosher and that meeting the criteria of the Islamic faith is termed halal.

For meat to be kosher, an animal must be killed in accordance with a method called shechita. Shechita slaughter rules state that animals must be killed humanely and to accomplish this an animal's throat must be cut with a sharp, smooth knife by a trained slaughterman, called a shochet. To be killed by the shechita method, an animal must be healthy and free of physical defects at the time of slaughter and it is these requirements which currently preclude the use of pre-slaughter stunning.

To produce halal meat, the permissibility of pre-slaughter stunning is less clearly prescribed. In order to be classed as halal, meat must come from an animal who was healthy and alive before the slaughter. In some Muslim communities, this is interpreted to mean that stunning is permissible, so long as the method does not cause physical damage or marked distress. Stunning is compulsory in New Zealand and halal red meat has been exported from New Zealand since the 1980s. Similarly, halal meat has been produced from stunned, as well as non-stunned, animals in several European countries including the UK. So it is possible for halal meat to have come from an animal who was stunned, and non-lethal electrical stunning is the most popular method.

Additionally, where pre-slaughter stunning has not been deemed permissible, stunning an animal immediately after their throat has been cut is allowed in some cases, to spare them protracted suffering.

The controversy surrounding slaughter without stunning arises from concerns that animals who have their throats cut while fully conscious experience unnecessary pain and suffering when otherwise widely utilized stunning methods are available to prevent this. The UK government's Farm Animal Welfare Committee (now Animal Welfare Committee) concluded that a large cut across the neck 'would result in very significant pain and distress in the period before insensibility supervenes' and cite research using electroencephalography (measurements of brain responses) to highlight that loss of consciousness typically takes 22–40 seconds in cattle, 5–7 seconds in sheep and is likely to take 20 seconds or more in poultry. There are differences between species because of differences in the blood supply to the brain. Cattle, for example, have vessels that still allow some blood to reach the brain (thereby keeping it alive and conscious for longer) even though their major neck vessels have been cut.

Ultimately, as the European Union's DIALREL (Dialogue on Issues of Religious Slaughter) project acknowledged, the controversy surrounding religious slaughter arises as a result of the apparent pitting of the human right to religious freedom against the growing global imperative for high standards of animal welfare. Respectful of the religious, cultural and political dimensions of this particular animal welfare problem, but with a professional mandate to prioritize the interests of animals, the British Veterinary Association (BVA) has led a longstanding campaign to improve animal welfare at the time of slaughter, including lobbying for an end to slaughter without pre-stunning in the UK. The Federation of Veterinarians of Europe holds the same position. Until such time as this goal is achieved, BVA is calling on the UK government to require clear labelling of meat from animals who have not been stunned before slaughter to enable consumer choice and for there to be a non-stun permit system, to ensure that the number of animals slaughtered without prior stunning does not exceed the relevant demand of the UK's religious communities. Such a permit is successfully employed in Germany and Austria, and the BVA says it should include a requirement for immediate post-cut stunning, to minimize suffering. The BVA also wants electrical waterbath stunning of poultry – the method I had observed – to be phased out, given its requirement for inversion and live-shackling of the birds and the risk of electroimmobilization, in which a bird is electrically immobilized but not stunned, so is still conscious when killed. It notes that many UK slaughterhouses have moved towards gas stunning of poultry, which eliminates this risk and minimizes the need for handling.

The BVA, together with a number of leading animal welfare charities, has had success in lobbying for mandatory closed-circuit television in abattoirs, which was introduced in England in 2018, followed by Scotland in 2021 and Wales announcing similar plans. The BVA is pressing for this across the UK's devolved nations as part of its inexhaustible efforts to ensure the lives of farmed animals end as humanely as possible.

We can all assist by informing and pressing our local politicians on these issues and, as ever, by purchasing food with packet logos that address our concerns – in this case, assuring that animals have been stunned before slaughter. Information on UK food labels that cover this is given in an appendix (see page 292).

My year's placements were complete, and snowfall had brought a hush to Formby's streets. Families were reuniting, and houses and pubs filled with warm Christmas Eve cheer. I padded through the snow to my former high school, where, together with a small team of volunteers and some charitable funding, we had created a small wildlife area, with a pond, nesting boxes and bird feeders. The school was deserted and I stood on the path we had carefully lain and looked around at the newly planted hazel, hawthorn and other trees and shrubs poking flimsily out of the snow. It was peaceful and pristine, a million miles from the noise and carnage of the abattoirs.

My binoculars, as always, hung around my neck, poised for use.

Usually, I use them to gain a better view of something that has caught my eye, but for some reason I began to casually scan around with them, gaining a more detailed perspective on the montage of jagged bark, bramble thorns and pine needles that scored hard, dark lines across the white surroundings. The wildlife area was bordered by the gardens of neighbouring houses and as my binoculars scanned slowly past a young rowan tree something registered deep within me; without thinking, I quickly reversed my direction to take a second look. This time lightning struck at my core. Perched within the branches of the berry-laden tree was a resplendent starling-sized bird I had never seen beyond the pages of a book. Pinkish-red with a plumed red crest sweeping from the back of their head, black eye mask and bib, and golden gilt-edging to their wings and tail, it was the most exotic-looking bird I had ever seen – a waxwing! I gripped my binoculars tightly as the bird moved towards the end of a branch, then nimbly swung down to extract berries, tossing them whole down their throat. As they did so, I was able to see the waxy red tips on their wing feathers that give the bird their name. Breeding in the remote northern pine forests of Scandinavia and Russia, waxwings, unlike regular migrants, fly to Western Europe only when crops of berries in their native lands are insufficient to sustain them. They therefore appear in the UK only in certain years, arriving in so-called irruptions.

Slowly recovering from the initial shock, I looked round to my right and saw a further six waxwings perched at the top of a tall poplar tree. Then, on a cold breeze, they alighted, sprinkling their tinkling calls like tiny finger bells across the silence. Christmas had come early.

CHAPTER 9

Skylarks and sheep

On Walney Island in Cumbria the spring air is dotted with the casual yelps of lesser black-backed and herring gulls as they drift towards their breeding colonies on invisible thermals. The sound evokes memories of dreamy summer days and intensifies to a raucous rabble at the colony itself, one of Europe's largest. On glistening pools and inlets, individuals from one of Europe's southernmost breeding colonies of eider ducks, famed for their insulating down, pass by in striking pied flotillas. Occasionally, groups of courting males toss back their heads and throw their rising 'ooo-oo' calls, like intrigued gossips, across to watching females and up to the grassy path where I am lying.

The nearby Cumbrian hills and moorlands are home to an estimated three million sheep, forming a mainstay of the local economy. Rams are typically put with the flocks of ewes in autumn, and lambs are tottering at their mothers' feet the following spring. The lambs live with their mothers out on the fields, sustained by milk and grass, until they are taken away to be slaughtered, at around five to eight months old, for the meat we simply call lamb.

The public's perception of sheep farming is generally favourable, with images of a naturalistic form of animal rearing that allows parent animals to live and mate naturally, then care for their young away from the confines and trappings of more intensive farming systems. Largely, this perception is accurate. Where sheep do not fare so well is in the public's perception of their intelligence. It was noted in Chapter 1 that the regard afforded to other species, and concern for their health and wellbeing, is often linked to their perceived intelligence. While it has been reiterated several times since that an animal does not need to be clever to suffer, if dismissing sheep as stupid runs the risk of diminishing concern for the welfare problems that they experience (some of which I will outline shortly), then the findings of Professor Keith Kendrick should first be noted. Kendrick is a neuroscientist who spent over 20 years studying the sensory and cognitive abilities of sheep at the Babraham Institute in Cambridge. His carefully controlled studies changed our understanding of how sheep think and experience the world, and challenged our widely held beliefs about them. As Kendrick writes,

> To many humans, sheep are regarded as being as close to an automaton and mindless animal species as can be imagined [...] as such, few give serious consideration to their welfare [...] What I will now outline about the cognitive, social and mental abilities of this species [...] will come as something of a shock to many, although hopefully less so to those who have spent considerable time looking after and interacting with sheep.

Kendrick notes that lowly opinions of the sheep mind are influenced by their tendency to be led rather than to lead and 'to adopt a safe group rather than an individual mentality'. However, the social group is very important to sheep, and some of Kendrick's early experiments examined the ways in which they communicate to one another using vocalizations. Most people recognize a sheep's bleating, but Kendrick revealed that the bleats we hear are more complex, and convey more information, than our human ears can discern. Using sound spectograms (graphs produced by recording equipment which analyses the structure of different sounds), it can first be seen that different individuals have different calls, allowing individuals to be identified and recognized by others. Bleats that sound the same to humans actually differ in content and structure depending on whether the sheep producing them is excited or stressed. A sheep with a low heart rate who becomes excited about the arrival of food makes a different bleat (though sounding the same to us) to one with a high heart rate who has been acutely stressed by a brief period of social isolation. In behavioural studies, sheep show a preference for bleats produced by excited rather than stressed individuals, lending support to the conclusion that they are able to distinguish between the two emotional states. It follows, as Kendrick explains, that sheep may be able to recognize that another sheep is experiencing stress or pain from their calls, and that this may be distressing for the sheep who is hearing such sounds.

Perhaps the studies that have stimulated the most interest in Keith Kendrick's work are those which have examined the facial recognition and memory capabilities of sheep. Kendrick and his research team devised experimental apparatus that allowed sheep to view video screens and to express their familiarity and preferences for different images by pressing panels to receive food. This experimental approach demonstrated that sheep can discriminate between at least 50 different sheep and 10 human faces at any one time. What is more, having learned to recognize these faces they then remember whether or not they were associated with food for at least several years. In 2001, these findings were published in the scientific journal *Nature*. Kendrick was also interested in the brain regions that are involved in such facial recognition and found that the main brain region for this capacity in people, the temporal cortex, is also the region where specialized cells for facial recognition are found in sheep.

Kendrick went on to investigate whether sheep can recognize different emotions being conveyed by facial expressions. Using images of the same sheep in calm and stressed states, and of the same humans with smiling and angry expressions, he found that by panel pressing to obtain food rewards, the sheep demonstrated clear preferences for rewards associated with smiling rather than angry humans and with sheep who were calm rather than those who had been stressed by isolation or shearing. In addition, despite having a general preference for familiar over unfamiliar sheep, they preferred to choose the face of a calm unfamiliar animal over a stressed familiar one.

Kendrick found that sheep are competent at facial recognition even when the individuals they are viewing (both sheep and human) are shown in profile, rather than face-on as they had originally been learned, suggesting that sheep can form a mental representation of an image and rotate it in their mind. Such a finding, as Kendrick points out, prompts intriguing and important questions about the nature of sheep consciousness, such as whether sheep may be capable of thinking about other individuals in their absence.

Sheep evolved in environments where the ground is dry, cold and stony, unlike the moist pastures where many commercial flocks now live. Modern-day pastures and husbandry practices can provide optimum conditions for certain bacteria to flourish and, as a result, foot infections and associated lameness are among the most serious problems affecting the health and wellbeing of farmed sheep.

Of the approximately 30 million sheep living in the United Kingdom, the UK government's Farm Animal Welfare Committee (FAWC, now Animal Welfare Committee) reported in 2011 that, with an estimated prevalence of around 10 per cent, there were likely to be approximately 3 million sheep lame at any one moment, equivalent to every single sheep in Cumbria. Sheep lameness in the UK is most commonly caused by the conditions of foot rot and contagious ovine digital dermatitis, both of which arise as a result of infection by bacteria. It is the painful inflammation, skin irritation and cell death caused by these bacteria which leave affected animals limping and hobbling around their fields.

In investigating the causes of the UK's sheep lameness problem, researchers confirmed that farmers are capable of recognizing lame sheep, but differences exist in their willingness or ability to catch and treat them. Allowing untreated lame sheep to endure pain or suffering is illegal in the UK; FAWC, in its report on sheep lameness, was firm in its view that the approach by some farmers, who never catch and treat lame sheep until the flock is gathered for some other reason, was 'unacceptable'. It also disadvantages the farmer, as delaying the identification and treatment of infectious causes of lameness allows those infections to spread more widely through the flock. Considering the various factors contributing to sheep lameness, FAWC concluded that much more should be done to minimize the condition – recognizing that some flocks achieve a prevalence of 2 per cent lameness – and that farmers and vets must work closely together to achieve this. In response, the five-point plan, based on five key aspects of sheep lameness control, was adopted as an agreed national strategy in 2014. Through concerted effort by vets and farmers, latest estimates have put the national prevalence in the UK flock at 3.2 per cent, while survey work has found that 72 per cent of farmers would now treat a lame sheep within three days of noticing them. With sustained focus, there is an optimism that FAWC's 2 per cent maximum prevalence target may be in sight.

Like most people, while out on country walks, I had seen cases of sheep struggling around fields, but I had had limited insight into some of the management practices employed by sheep farmers when their flocks are handled and housed. One of the key developments in safeguarding lamb welfare had been the housing of ewes at lambing time, to protect the vulnerable lambs from chilling and predation. In mid-March I took a train from Liverpool to Exeter to spend a month assisting on a sheep farm at its busy lambing time.

The farmhouse was set deep in the Devon countryside and had recently invested in a large, new lambing shed, which enjoyed a commanding view across the surrounding fields. Simon, a university classmate, and I had both made the journey to undertake the placement together and having unpacked our belongings in the family home, we were taken by the farmer, Patrick, up the gravelly path to the shed.

Stepping inside for the first time, we heard the occasional shuffle of straw from beneath the heaving fleeces of over a hundred heavily pregnant ewes in an otherwise strangely quiet building. During mating the previous autumn, rams on the farm had been raddled, meaning that when they mounted a ewe, a coloured mark was left on her fleece. This, together with ultrasound scanning, meant that pregnancies on the farm had been closely monitored and the ewes were organized in the shed according to predicted due dates, while recent mothers were individually penned with their frail and endearing newborns.

Patrick reminded us of signs of impending birth and advised us of the circumstances in which our assistance for a ewe might be required. Less than a week later, I was up in the lambing shed on my own, having left Simon with the farmer and his family to rest and sleep after another well-received farmhouse supper.

I became familiar with the sight of ewes in the main pen separating from the rest of the group and becoming restless, pawing at the ground to create a birthing area. The hush in the warm shed would be broken by the sound of their distinctive pre-birth bleats and I would monitor from a safe distance to check that their straining was productive and the lambs were passed within a safe timeframe. The first time that I suspected a problem, I managed to correctly identify a malpresentation with my fastidiously scrubbed hand, but was unable to confidently judge just how firm I could be to correct it and summoned Patrick from his bed for assistance. But as the nights passed, I gained experience and confidence in creating a mental image of the presentation at my fingertips and making necessary adjustments to the unborn lamb's positioning to allow them to pass. Intervention was kept to an absolute minimum, but it was satisfying to carefully ease a slippery neonate from the protective world of their struggling mother, remove mucus and remnants of her life-giving membranes from their mouth and nostrils with my finger, and see her lick the helpless animal clean in a dimly lit shed beneath the stars.

During the day, as well as helping with the lambing, Simon and I assisted with general jobs and duties on and around the farm. These included assembling pens for the ewes and their lambs, repairing hay mangers and, again – the norm it seemed on farm placements – 'mutilating' the young animals without anaesthesia or pain relief.

In the case of the lambs, the task in hand was to remove their tails and testicles. While Simon slept in preparation for his night shift, Patrick, a driven man who had followed in his father's sheep-farming footsteps, furnished me with the information and equipment I would need to perform the procedures efficiently. He was well-spoken and punctilious in his delivery.

'OK, Sean, I know you haven't done this before but it's not difficult. You're just going to put two of these rings on, one on the tail and one around the scrotum, with this device.'

Patrick brandished the device, a so-called elastrator, in his right hand. It resembled a pair of stainless steel pliers with four short projections at the opening end. The rings, filling a small, clear plastic bag, were approximately a centimetre and a half in diameter and made of thick rubber. One of the rings was placed over the four projections and when the elastrator handles were pressed together, the ring stretched open in readiness to receive an appendage.

Patrick picked up a one-day-old lamb and held him against his thighs with the lamb's feet facing forwards. He took a ring from the bag, placed it over the elastrator and collected the lamb's small scrotum into his left hand. Having checked that both testicles were present, he used the elastrator to pass the stretched ring over the scrotum and then released the pressure on the handles, allowing the rubber ring to close tightly across the neck of the scrotum, where it joins the lamb's body. He deftly slid the ring off the elastrator's projections and, with a swift action, moved the elastrator away leaving the rubber ring in place.

'They'll drop off in ten days or so,' he said matter-of-factly, gesturing towards the testicles.

Patrick placed the lamb back down on the straw and applied a second rubber ring to the elastrator.

'Could you pick him up for me again, please, Sean?'

I scooped the lamb back up, who wriggled and bleated for a few moments in my arms, then oriented the lamb's back end towards Patrick. He opened the elastrator's jaws for a second time, and this time moved the ring along the lamb's woolly tail.

'The important thing here is to make sure you leave enough tail behind to cover the anus, and the vulva in females,' said Patrick, demonstrating as he spoke. Then, with a similarly swift movement, he removed the elastrator, leaving the constricting ring in place. 'That should drop off within a couple of weeks,' he said.

We spent the next couple of hours repeating the procedures and by the end of the morning I had castrated and tail docked around 20 lambs with increasing ease.

As with most management practices associated with large groups of animals on farms, whether vaccinating, administering preventive anti-parasitic medication or removing tails, we had had to proceed efficiently throughout the morning, quickly replacing one lamb with the next. Each was returned to the pen with their mother, but it was not until the end of the castrating and tail docking session, when Patrick had gathered up his belongings and returned to the farmhouse, that I was able to take a few minutes to watch the most recently manipulated lambs in the pen next to me.

I focussed on one lamb in particular, who was the last to be handled and returned to the pen. The lamb's movement seemed stilted and cautious. He rose slowly to his feet, wagging his tail stump vigorously, then quickly dropped his back end down onto the straw and slowly lowered his front end. He lay still for a moment, then shuffled and kicked out with his back legs. After a few seconds, he slowly stood up again and resumed flicking his tail. He shifted position, struggled to his feet, then collapsed down on to the straw. His mother repeatedly sniffed and licked him, and pawed at the straw close to him, as his sides rose and fell with rapid breaths. I continued watching for a few minutes as the lamb's pattern of rising, collapsing and kicking repeated, before joining the others in the farmhouse.

Simon and I bade farewell to the farm as the first returning swallows began streaming their tales of Saharan adventure around the buildings and fields. I journeyed north, back to Liverpool, and the late afternoon sun strobed orange through my dozing eyelids as Devon grew ever-distant.

As for castration and tail docking in piglets, and disbudding in calves, scientific research into the pain experienced by lambs being castrated and tail docked has made valuable use of behavioural and physiological indicators, such as the behaviours I had witnessed, and elevations in the stress hormone, cortisol. The administration of local anaesthesia helps to validate these indicators and its effects can be observed on the YouTube channel of the EU-funded Animal Welfare Indicators project. On short video clips of lamb behaviour following tail docking and castration, there are clearly observable differences between siblings who have been mutilated with and without local anaesthesia, as the medicated lamb in each clip lies still while the other shifts and kicks restlessly under the watch of their attentive mother. This acute pain typically lasts for around two hours, then is followed by further inflammation and pain which can persist for more than 48 hours. Separate studies have confirmed that ewes are more attentive to their lambs when they are experiencing pain, and measurably more so than when their lambs have simply experienced stress (such as social isolation). Researcher Dr Sophie Hild and her colleagues were unable to conclude that a ewe's maternal care in these circumstances helps to mitigate the pain of their lamb, but comment that 'the possibility that such a phenomenon occurs later cannot be ruled out'. In the light of Keith Kendrick's findings, retaining an open mind on such emotional possibilities seems wise.

Several million lambs are castrated each year in the UK and many more are tail docked. Legislation prohibits the use of rubber elastrator rings beyond the age of seven days, though there is no evidence to support the suggestion that lambs feel less pain during their first week of life.

As in the case of other mutilations applied to farmed animals, benefits are believed to accrue for both farmers (or the markets they supply) and the animals themselves. In the case of castration, these include the prevention of indiscriminate breeding between mixed flocks of sexually active male and female lambs (which could lead to lambs being born with little chance of survival); market demand for certain carcass characteristics associated with being castrated; and avoiding fighting and injury that can occur between uncastrated males. For tail docking, the cited benefit is the prevention of a condition called fly strike. With this condition, flies are attracted to soiled fur around the animal's rear end. Here they lay their eggs which hatch out into maggots. The maggots then begin eating the animal's flesh, causing painful tissue damage and ultimately death. The presence of a long woolly tail dangling around the anus can increase the amount of faecal material that accumulates there, increasing the young animal's attractiveness to the flies that could imperil them.

It was late when I returned to my parents' home in Formby but it felt good to be back, with the prospect of enjoying some more of the spring. After my month away I had planned to have a long, re-energizing sleep extending far into the following morning, but I awoke at 5:15am to a chorus of coal tits, wrens, robins, blackbirds and chaffinches singing close to my bedroom window. A woodpigeon joined in, and I sat up on my bed and watched as the portly bird lowered his head and leaned forward, as though facing into a strong wind. With a look of determination, he heaved his shoulders, pumped his tail and expanded his throat as his loud cooing echoed with the might of his wooded world. The sun was shining and my mind turned to the dewy farmland at Cabin Hill. Fifteen minutes later I had tied my bicycle to a fence and was crossing the quiet railway line on the footpath there, leading to the beach.

The path stretching ahead was empty and the early haze was slowly disappearing from the open fields as the day began to warm. For as many springs as I can remember, two wild performances have found their stage in the country skies around the Cabin Hill National Nature Reserve. Nature's rhythms provide an anchor line, threading through time like a guiding rope. Despite farmland birds having declined more severely than those in any other habitat, with a fall of 54 per cent in the UK since

1970, I still somehow cling to a certainty that on this path, on a sunny spring morning, I will experience the spectacle of displaying skylarks and lapwings.

I walk with the dark strip of young pine trees screening out the rifle range on my left, and then, from high above the ploughed field ahead, a faint hurrying stream of piccolo notes meets me on the path. They infiltrate me with their hypnotic constancy and pull me closer until I am beneath my first singing skylark of the spring, transfixed and seared by his merciless beam of joyful optimism. The bird bubbles through his chosen champagne sky, fluting vertically high above his territory. As a spider conjures a web from its liquid silk, so the singing skylark, producing multiple notes a second, weaves an imaginary chord from his, hauling himself up it higher and higher until it is barely possible to detect him as a speck in the sky above. And still he sings. The energy, rapidity and unpredictability of his song are mesmerizing and helter-skelter around the DNA of every cell in my body. The bird lifts on endlessly beating wings, occasionally pausing before his next determined ascent. In a woodland, tens of species would be pouring their song into the fresh morning air, but above farmland, equivalent expectation and ability musters from 360 degrees of open sky and channels through the throat of a single sparrow-sized chorister with the ferocity of a great whale's blow. The skylark's ascent resuscitates the winter-wearied countryside. Red admirals make territorial sallies in woodland glades while ponds and pools fill with reflections of emerging foliage. Between each pause of the bird's reviving song flight, flushes of colour return to the hedgerows and delicate eyelashes of Queen Anne's lace flutter in the country lanes as the land reawakens. At the peak of his ascent, the skylark spreads his wings one last time and parachutes to earth enshrouded by the dazzling apparel of his unfaltering music. Once he is on the ground, I watch through binoculars as he looks around, seeking the approval of an unrevealed choreographer. A nearby reed bunting emits his single-note song, resigned to life in a lyrical hinterland.

The military rifle range has been managed sympathetically for skylarks, and three more birds take to the sky in turn, like ornamental fountains, ensuring that my morning walk is filled with bird song from the moment I arrive to the moment I leave. I sit down on a grassy tussock next to the footpath and look out across the ploughed furrows, laid out like a maestro's blank stave. The skylarks pour their inexhaustible tremolos from the dizzying ledger lines, but to my right, the sliding notes of a swanee whistle bounce and dip through the awakening sky; mapping a course for their plumed soloist whose May Day ribbons of black, white, rich chestnut and green-purple iridescence twist a colourful treble clef across the stirring score. A lapwing tumbles and calls on his display flight, displacing the sky with his paddle-like wings: three flaps to the left, three flaps to the right. At a distance he looks strikingly black and white, curling through the sky like a ribbon pulled across a scissor blade. But then I watch through binoculars and see the sunlight picking out the chestnut beneath his tail and the shimmering colours on his back. His flight is extraordinary, like a bird possessed. He zigzags, producing an ethereal hum from specially modified feathers on his wings, then he begins to climb with his legs dangling. Next, his head and neck recoil sharply twice as he emits a double motif of his peculiar pure song, then makes a third wheezy offering as he enters a vertical stoop towards the field. The skylark's notes, dancing on the earth like falling rain, lift him to immediately repeat his performance from the beginning.

I continue walking down the path. The planting of the pine trees along it has allowed red squirrels to extend their range from the nearby pinewoods and I stop in my tracks when a branch ahead bows more deeply and aggressively than the breeze can push it. A red squirrel emerges onto an exposed branch and appears not to notice me as he begins determinedly ordering his glowing fur with precise tongue strokes. Soon the world around me will be bustling, but I am blissfully removed for just a little while longer as an invisible observer.

I reflect on the lambs. Could the natural freedoms enjoyed by the sheep and their young extend to being spared their painful manipulations, despite the proffered justifications?

The worst reason for continuing would appear to be because we have always done it. As the UK nations' Sheep Welfare Codes point out, 'Farmers and shepherds should consider carefully whether castration [and tail docking are] necessary within any particular flock.'

To reduce the requirement for castration, the British Veterinary Association and the UK's Sheep Veterinary Society recommend that management practices aimed at achieving slaughter weight prior to sexual maturity should be adopted whenever possible. Where sexual maturity is reached before slaughter, they say that breeding activity should be prevented by physical and visual separation of ram lambs from ewe lambs.

The benefit of tail docking to some sheep, by preventing debilitating fly strike, is recognized, although it is not straightforward weighing this against the pain caused to all of the lambs, many of whom would not have developed fly strike. Although tail docking may reduce faecal soiling around a lamb's back end, other approaches can also reduce this, such as effective parasite control (thereby preventing diarrhoea), shearing the wool of the tail and around the anus (sometimes called crutching) and selecting breeds with an open fleece that creates less humidity at the skin surface and so is less attractive to flies. There are currently no analgesics and a limited number of anaesthetics licensed for use in sheep within the UK, which reduces the potential for their use. The medicine Meloxicam provides significant pain relief to sheep, and products containing it have been licensed for use in sheep in Canada and Australia. So, in addition to these preventive recommendations, the veterinary associations – and FAWC, when they reported on lamb castration and tail docking in 2008 – are clear that, for as long as both mutilations are considered to be necessary, the UK government and industry must develop and authorize a local anaesthetic and analgesic protocol for use in field conditions, to alleviate the pain being felt by the millions of lambs subjected to these procedures each year. Growing numbers of farmers are taking a three Rs approach to mutilations, supported and assisted by their vets – replacing the need to perform them through alternative approaches, reducing the numbers of animals affected to the minimum necessary and refining the procedures through increased use of pain relief. Government and industry are more likely to accelerate this welcome progress if they feel it to be the pressing will of us all, as citizens and consumers.

Spring boils with new life and, having started my day early at Cabin Hill, in the evening I visit Ainsdale National Nature Reserve. I watch from the Coastal Road as a globe sun sinks slowly towards the Irish Sea. I am alone in the gradually darkening dunes as the air cools and I feel the dampening ground through my trousers as I sit next to a moist dune slack.

In the morning, the sun will rise and life will shine again from every nook and cranny. Blackcaps visibly shake as they belt out their pure, warbling songs from hedgerows and thickets. As I sit outside at a wooden table, the peace is intermittently interrupted by the quiet rasping of wasps harvesting tiny mouthfuls of wood for their nests. A blackbird who approaches from the lawn, closer and closer, taps a Morse code greeting on the paved patio as he pecks up a welcome meal of ants.

Now, the sound I have been waiting for begins to float up around me from the dusky dunes. It is a long reeling sound that repeats in steady pulses. Some of it is coming from the shallow pool which I am crouched next to, but when I stand up there are echoes all around me as a host of calls emanate from a specially protected network of similar scrapes that extend in a corridor throughout the dunes. It is the sound of Europe's loudest amphibian – locally known as the Birkdale nightingale (after the nearby village of Birkdale) – and one of the UK's most endangered. As they emerge from sandy hibernation burrows where they have survived the winter, I am now surrounded by one of the UK's largest-surviving populations of natterjack toads, with males calling enthusiastically to attract females. Without causing disturbance, I can see one in the shallow margin of the pool, his presence revealed by the gently rippling waves created by his impressive inflating and deflating throat sack. The sack is blue tinged, while a distinctive yellow stripe runs from between his yellow-green eyes and through the knobbly green-and-red-tinged landscape of his short back, no longer than my thumb. The calls pulse all around me in the darkness and I think back to the morning skylarks valiantly pumping life into the surrounding countryside. I close my eyes and listen. The sounds merge together in my mind until I am tuned in to the unified beating heart of the dunes. I have heard, today, some of nature's finest and most celebrated wild musicians, and the toads' finale heralds that spring is, once again, well and truly alive. I have tuned in to rhythms as old as life on earth and the reassuring sound continues to beat steadily, both within the dunes and deep within me, as I finally concede my day's end and leave the coast for home.

CHAPTER 10

Hummingbirds and horses

My university supervisors had suggested that my foray into caged zebra finch welfare might be of interest at the congress of the International Society for Applied Ethology in California – for scientists using behaviour to assess animal welfare. I was yet to fulfil my placement requirement with horses and was accepted by a veterinary clinic in the San Francisco Bay region, which I would attend when the congress ended. For the first few days, I couldn't get over the size of the Californian roads – or the size of my breakfasts. The golden towers of the city's famous bridge were spyhopping out of daily summer fogs that rolled in from the Pacific. Alcatraz sat ominously to its east while Pier 39 bore the tonnage of the Bay's wild Californian sea lions.

The congress was held at the University of California in Davis. In the breaks I explored the 100-acre campus arboretum, where 3.5 miles of paths looped through carefully tended horticultural collections and along the banks of the Putah Creek. The waterway is crossed by a series of bridges and as I walked beneath the California Avenue Bridge I became aware of the chattering and clicks of roosting bats within gaps in the concrete, a foot or so above my head. A small interpretation sign revealed that they were insect-eating bats called Yuma myotis and I returned to the quiet arboretum later to watch them dropping into the dusky night.

The following morning, I was drawn back to the arboretum. It had a recorded list of over 135 species of birds and one I was keen to see in particular. Never before had I seen a hummingbird, or perhaps even imagined that I ever would. But the arboretum was home to one species – Anna's hummingbird – and I set off at dawn with the heady notion that I might be able to find one. On the way, a postcard caught my eye in the window of the university gift shop. An artistic image of a red chilli on a white background, with a pair of green leaves either side, composed to look like a hovering hummingbird. I thought I would buy one as a quirky souvenir, but then thought again. I would buy one if I saw a real hummingbird.

I set off along a path towards an area that became increasingly wooded with looming conifers. There had been plenty of scarlet blooms along the way to attract hungry hummingbirds, but as I became increasingly surrounded by the trees it felt as though I was moving further away from likely hummingbird habitat. Then ahead I could see the path open into a clearing and music was emanating from a small wooden hut. Rage Against the Machine has an angry, thrashing quality. This early in the morning, the arboretum was devoid of people and the track selection seemed slightly improbable.

'Heey!'

A voice called down from the veranda and I looked up to see a man leaning casually against the balcony. He had cropped black hair and a tight T-shirt tucked into dark jeans.

'How's it going, man?' His voice was deep. To the left of the hut was a motorbike and a stereo placed on the ground.

'Good, thanks.'

'You been here before?' he asked.

'No, I'm just here for a walk.'

He saw me looking at a drinking fountain behind him on the veranda.

'Thirsty? Come up here,' he exclaimed, smiling. 'That's the finest water in the whole of America!'

'Cheers.' I hesitated, then cautiously ascended the wooden steps. The lyrics to 'Calm Like a Bomb' spewed out of the stereo. I let the cool water arc into my mouth while keeping the man in my peripheral vision.

'That was good,' I said, wiping my mouth with the back of my hand.

'Yeah, it's good,' he said, still smiling, and with an unnerving habit of looking past me as though watching to see if anyone else was around. 'What's your name?'

'Sean.'

'I'm Pete.'

'Do you spend much time here?' I asked.

He gave a gravelly chuckle. 'No way, man! I'm from the east coast. Just out of prison yesterday and finding my direction, you know what I'm saying?' The word 'Ignite!' bawled out of the stereo nine times and funnelled up through the trees into the sky above.

I started to slowly reverse down the steps and Pete followed. For some reason I didn't want to take my eyes off him. I was glad I hadn't met him when I was looking for bats the night before. He fixed his gaze on the binoculars around my neck.

'You lookin' for something special?'

'Yeah, hummingbirds.'

'Ahh,' he said, tilting his head back. He smiled again. 'That'd be real nice.'

'Have you ever seen one?' I asked.

He paused before replying. 'I've seen a lot of things in my time.'

This time it was my turn to notice something beyond him. A tiny movement in some branches behind Pete, about 20 feet from the ground. I tried to keep Pete in my field of vision, but was distracted. There was something in the tree.

The stereo reached the end of its final track and the clearing fell silent. As our ears adjusted, a new sound could be heard, pricking the area where I had seen movement. It was high pitched and scratchy, tuneless but intricate. I scanned the evergreen fronds but it was hopeless without my binoculars. I ignored Pete for a moment and raised them to my eyes.

On an exposed branch, the silhouette of a long, thin bill added to the pine needle mosaic against the blue sky. My gathering awe discharged through the tiny bird's bill, igniting a glistening plumage of emerald and rose-pink. An Anna's hummingbird; I could see his throat moving as he sang.

'Check this out!' I said excitedly to Pete.

'You got one?'

'Yeah, have a look if you want!' I pulled the strap of the binoculars over my head and thrust them towards him. He pointed them at the tree and turned the focus wheel.

'OK, I got that. Cool.' For a moment my apprehension passed as I shared this momentous experience with a stranger. Hummingbirds were exotic: birds of wildlife documentaries, with their brilliantly decorated tininess and precise blurred flight. Then I noticed the time – the congress was about to begin.

'It was good to meet you. Thanks for the water.'

'You got it.'

I retraced my steps quickly back through the arboretum. My cheeks had a red chilli flush when I arrived at the gift shop and bought the postcard.

I took a thundering Amtrak train from Davis and began my placement with the equine practice. We were on our way to a horse yard where the vet, Richard, had warned me of the conditions we might find.

'The place stinks,' he drawled. 'There're flies everywhere, so keep the windows up. Ted's a funny fella, so you're best just listening to me.' Our truck's wheels whipped up a trail of dust as we pulled onto the yard. There were three pigs in an unshaded pen and two dogs barking in another.

We were there to see a horse with a history of a foot abscess. Richard had seen improvement treating the horse with a former owner, but the animal had recently been bought by Ted and apparently the hoof had deteriorated badly. After a clinical assessment, Richard confirmed that it was in a poor way and would need further treatment.

He needed to return to his truck for his equipment. 'I'll be back in a minute,' he said, as he walked off across the yard. I followed Ted into a nearby barn to shelter from the hot sun.

I guessed that Ted was in his fifties. He was a heavy man and seemed to find breathing difficult. He collapsed down into a flimsy wooden chair, with a partly buttoned check shirt resting on his belly. I stood opposite him, leaning against the bottom half of a stable door.

'So, how y'enjoyin' California then, kid?'

'It's really good,' I answered. 'I really like San Francisco.'

He nodded and moved his stubbly jaw up and down as he chewed slowly on some gum.

Some similar pleasantries followed, but we were both distracted by a foal in the stable behind me, who had noticed the human addition to his living space and had taken to mouthing inquisitively at my collar. I smiled at Ted with a paternal delight. Ted stared back at me and looked at the young animal over my shoulder, as he had been during our exchanges. Then he put his hands on the arms of his chair and pushed himself upwards.

He strode straight towards me with an angry look on his face, then raised his right arm and pulled it backwards with a tightly clenched fist. Thinking he was going to punch me in the face, I ducked to the side as his large arm flew towards me and landed his curled knuckles, like a wrecking ball, on the foal's sensitive nose. The foal whinnied loudly and recoiled to the back of his stable. Ted shuffled back to his chair with an air of a job well done and sank back down into it.

'You gotta' treat them like that early,' he said, emphasizing the 'gotta'. There was a short pause. 'You married?'

'No,' I replied indignantly, my heart still thumping with the sense of a near miss and anger at what I'd seen.

'Sometimes you've gotta' treat your women like that too.' He beamed at me with squinting eyes, as though satisfied to be passing on such useful life lessons.

I walked out of the barn.

Animals experience differing kinds of harms at the hands of people. On the one hand, through ignorance, they may not have their basic care needs met: for example, suitable food, healthcare and appropriate companionship. Recall from Chapter 1 that the UK's Animal Welfare Acts introduced a legal duty of care to ensure that a kept animal's Five Welfare Needs are met. But deliberate cruelty is different. It is now an offence not to care for animals properly, but to inflict intentional cruelty is still punishable under UK law, as it has been for over a century.

Ted's comment raised another important concern. In situations where individuals behave abusively towards animals, they may also be abusive towards other vulnerable members of their household. In some cases, violence is practised on animals before moving on to human victims. In other cases, abuse of animals is used as a means of threat or intimidation.

The UK's Links Group is a group of organizations from animal welfare, child protection, domestic violence, local government, veterinary and human medical backgrounds who promote the welfare and safety of vulnerable children, adults and animals. They provide invaluable guidance and education to veterinary and other healthcare professionals about the link between abuse of these different groups, recognizing signs of non-accidental injury and providing materials on how to report concerns while complying with professional responsibilities towards client confidentiality. In short, they ensure people like me know how to act when confronted by future situations like this one. As the group explains:

It is well known that abuse through neglect or maltreatment is perpetrated in a number of relationships: child maltreatment, domestic violence, animal abuse and abuse of older people.

Increasingly it has come to be recognized that there are complex interrelationships within these abnormal relationships. For instance, children that are abusive to animals may have themselves been abused or if serious animal abuse is occurring, other forms of domestic or family violence may also be present. Refuges for women are familiar with the situation of desperate women reluctant to leave their violent homes because of threats to their beloved pets. Threats or actual harm to pets or other animals may be used to ensure silence over the abuse to children and vulnerable adults including the elderly.

The Links Group provides distressing anecdotal evidence, gathered by police forces, of the link between domestic abuse and animal abuse. For example:

- A male perpetrator of domestic abuse bought a dog for his wife. During an argument he took the dog into the kitchen and killed the dog by cutting their throat. He went on to become a convicted serial murderer and rapist.

- During a historic investigation of child abuse, it was established that the abuser had over a number of years physically and sexually abused his wife and their children. All the witnesses spoke of a great deal of animal cruelty including microwaving cats and cutting dogs' heads off with spades.

- During a violent domestic incident, the perpetrator threw boiling water over his partner and then tried to strangle her. He then picked up a large kitchen knife, called the children into the room and killed two pet finches by stabbing them to death in front of the children.

There are many reasons for protecting and promoting animal welfare, but where deliberate cruelty is concerned, protection of human wellbeing and safety is one of them.

Some deliberate abuses of animals are administered for the purpose of improving animal performances, for human entertainment. Of the world's estimated 60 million or so horses, the vast majority in the developed world are used for human recreation or sport. In California, on rounds with one of the younger vets, Carly, we stopped for a break at one of the stable yards and she told me of some of the practices she and fellow graduates had encountered in the US during their short careers.

Gingering, she told me, is a practice whereby ginger – a mild chemical irritant – is inserted into the anus or vagina of some Arab horses to encourage them to hold their tail high in the show ring.

Tail nicking, also practised in the world of showing, is performed on some Saddlebred and Tennessee Walking Horses to artificially raise their tails. It involves cutting tendons on the underside of the tail, then placing the tail in a harness to prevent it from gradually sinking down. The harness may be worn most of the time when the horse is not being ridden. Horses cannot be let out unsupervised when wearing the harness, so are individually stabled.

A third example, to achieve a high-stepping gait called the Big Lick in shown Tennessee Walking Horses, involves the application of caustic substances or a mechanical device to a horse's front feet, in a practice called soring. Substances such as mustard oil are brushed into the horse's feet, which are then bandaged to improve absorption. The resulting pain causes the horse to shift their weight to their back feet and lift their front feet higher than usual to minimize their contact time with the ground. During training, metal weights are tied around the front feet so that, as they bang against the sensitized skin, the pain is increased and the foot-lifting response is further exaggerated. Disturbing undercover video footage of this practice can be viewed on the Humane Society US YouTube video, 'Tennessee Walking Horse Investigation Exposes Cruelty'.

Referring to practices such as these, Dr Jim Heird, Executive Professor and Coordinator of the Equine Initiative at Texas A&M University and a past Chairman of the American Quarter Horse Association Judges Committee, wrote in 2011 that 'Inhumane treatment has become a part of the show horse industry in the USA [...] No breed or show group is free of practices that the general public would find distasteful or unacceptable.' He reported, however, that many practices were now receiving attention from the showing industry. The American Association of Equine Practitioners (AAEP), the American Veterinary Medical Association (AVMA) and the Humane Society Veterinary Medical Association have condemned the 'cruel, inhumane, unethical and illegal practice of soring' and are lobbying the US Congress to pass the Prevent All Soring Tactics (PAST) Act. In 2015, backed by the AVMA, the AAEP also condemned 'the alteration of the tail of the horse for cosmetic or competitive purposes', including nicking. In 2021 a concerned US veterinary specialist wrote that unethical tail procedures undertaken for the show ring are still 'alarmingly widespread'.

As always, the role for us all, as aware and concerned citizens, is recognized, with Dr Heird noting that 'Some of [the] new efforts are due to the negative publicity received concerning these practices, and some are a proactive response by the organisations to the increased awareness the public has of inhumane practices.'

I was shocked to hear of Carly's experiences and looked over at the horses housed in a long row of stables across the yard. I had enjoyed visiting stables at various times during my life, especially on dark winter evenings when dim lights, draped tack, the evocative smells of feed and fur, and the animals' quiet nickering could colour gentle encounters with a Dickensian nostalgia. But aside from the acts of cruelty I had witnessed and heard about, how do these sensitive animals fare, living variously between the confines of their stables, exercise areas and the various show grounds, race tracks and myriad other destinations where their human purposes are realized? Do we meet their physical and psychological needs, despite the large amount of money, attention and love often lavished upon them? As I wondered, I watched the long nose of one of the horses swaying from side to side over her stable door like a wiper blade, an action she had barely stopped doing since we arrived.

As with other animals discussed in this book, today's domesticated horses remain similar to their wild ancestors. Despite being under the care of humans, they remain physically, physiologically and behaviourally adapted to the open grassland plains in which they evolved. As with all domesticated animals, we have taken control of horses, selectively breeding them for our work and, latterly, leisure purposes. But this constitutes a vanishingly small period in the horse's evolutionary history . The many feral populations of horses around the world (domestic horses who have returned to a free-living, wild state) demonstrate that their behaviour, including their social and foraging behaviour, has changed very little in their approximately 6,000 years of domestication.

The horse of the open plains is a prey animal, with their independently movable ears and near-360-degree vision attuned to the approach of possible predators. Group living allows for more pairs of eyes to detect danger and reduces the risk of any individual horse being caught and killed. With enough advance warning, they will run like wild horses; otherwise they will fight and kick with their legs, in close combat. Whether free-living or domesticated, horses will naturally spend up to 16 hours out of every 24 foraging and grazing, and rarely choose to fast for more than four hours at a time.

Despite this, the way we choose to feed, house and manage today's horses exposes them to living conditions that are very different to those of their wild ancestors. Most horses are confined in stables for varying lengths of time (sometimes near permanently), are often not housed together and are fed a diet containing high levels of cereals and low levels of roughage, with long periods of fasting between meals. The horse's digestive system and behaviour are adapted for very different conditions, so how does this affect them?

We are accustomed to the sights of meticulously groomed and braided show jumpers or the sleek sheen of elite equine athletes at racecourses, tended by teams of devoted grooms and trainers. Many people would be surprised to learn that many of these horses are afflicted with stomach ulcers linked to the unnatural lifestyles that they lead. In fact, over a third of pleasure horses may have a stomach (or gastric) ulcer, over half of show horses and a high 80 to 100 per cent of racehorses in training.

Gastric ulcers are open sores in the lining of the stomach which, in people, cause a burning or gnawing pain. In equine gastric ulcer syndrome, five grades of ulcer severity are recognized, diagnosed by passing an endoscope (fibre optic camera) into a horse's stomach. In Grade 0 the stomach lining is healthy. In Grade 1, the stomach lining is intact, but areas are reddened and inflamed; in Grade 2, small ulcers are visible; in Grade 3, larger ulcers are visible; and in Grade 4, there are extensive ulcers, some merging with each other, creating areas of deep ulceration. Different grades are expected to cause different levels of pain, ranging from a persistent low level of pain causing signs such as a poor appetite, to more severe pain causing horses to grind their teeth, show signs of colic and react with discomfort when a girth (saddle strap) is tightened.

One of the key factors associated with gastric ulcers in horses is that the foods we feed, and the intervals at which we feed them, are mismatched to the horse's digestive system. Because horses have evolved to graze on grasslands, their digestive system became adapted to digest frequent small amounts of nibbled grass and vegetation. Stomach acid in both humans and horses breaks down our food so that nutrients can be released and absorbed. In meal-eating humans, this acid is released only when we eat, but in horses, acid is released continually, in readiness for the steady trickle of food. In the wild state, this acid is absorbed and buffered by the fibrous stomach contents. But in domestic horses, fed intermittent high-energy, cereal-based meals, and relatively small quantities of hay, the acid gradually accumulates in the stomach.

Additionally, food intake stimulates saliva production. Saliva is alkaline, so when horses graze naturally they produce a steady flow of alkaline saliva which helps to neutralize their stomach acid. But when they are stabled and fed periodic high-energy, low-fibre meals each day, saliva production is not stimulated in the periods between meals, resulting in insufficient saliva in the stomach to neutralize the acid.

Equine gastric ulceration can also be linked to stressors such as training and transport. The prevalence of gastric ulcers in both racing and endurance horses nearly doubles during the competitive period compared to the out-of-competition period.

As equine veterinary specialists point out, gastric ulcers, occurring at a 'distressingly high prevalence', are 'often a man-made disease'. So why don't we feed horses diets that are more suited to their digestive physiology?

Partly, it is because we stable horses, restricting their access to pasture. They may be provided with hay in a net, but this is typically eaten swiftly and their fibre intake is still reduced. More importantly, the performance demands that we place on many horses mean that, for many, they cannot meet their training demands and sporting targets if only powered by grass.

My colleagues in equine veterinary practice may be resigned to making futile therapeutic recommendations: for example 'removal of horses from training and turning them out to pasture appears to be a very effective means of therapy in many cases; of course, this is frequently not possible for working horses'. Many horses, especially racehorses, are maintained on an ongoing preventive dose of medication that suppresses their production of stomach acid. The governing body of equestrian activities such as dressage, show jumping and eventing permits this drug to be used during competition, as long as its use is declared, while the British Horseracing Authority does not.

One of the possible ways that some horses may try to alleviate the pain and discomfort of gastric ulcers is to repeatedly bite on hard surfaces in their living environment: an example of stereotypic behaviour – abnormal repetitive behaviour – called crib biting. Crib biting has been reported as being performed by up to 10.5 per cent of captive domestic horses. The behaviour involves grasping a fixed object (often the stable door) with the incisor teeth, contracting the lower neck muscles, drawing air into the first part of the oesophagus and, in so doing, emitting a characteristic grunt. A horse who has developed crib biting may spend from 15 to 65 per cent of their time doing it, every day.

Using endoscopy to examine the stomachs of crib-biting versus non-crib-biting foals revealed that the crib-biting foals' stomachs were significantly more inflamed and ulcerated. The foals were then randomly allocated to a control (normal) diet, or a diet containing antacid. After three and a half months, and a repeat of the endoscopic examination, there was a significant improvement in the condition of the stomachs where the antacid diet had been fed, and the crib-biting foals in this group also showed the greatest decline in crib-biting behaviour. It has been proposed that at least part of the reason why some horses repeatedly bite at the fixtures and fittings in their living environment may be to stimulate saliva production and neutralize the stomach acid that is causing them discomfort, though this has not been confirmed. Instead, subsequent researchers have concluded that both gastric ulcers and crib biting may simply be linked to the horses' 'environmental and physiological stress'.

The horse who was repetitively swaying their head over their stable door was also exhibiting a stereotypy called weaving. Other stereotypies in captive horses include box walking (or stall walking) and wind sucking.

Box walking involves repetitively pacing within a stable, while wind sucking is similar to crib biting but without grasping onto a solid object. Stereotypies have traditionally been called 'vices' by horse owners, but this has connotations of a bad, nuisance-causing habit, rather than a sign of an underlying problem requiring consideration of the horse's wellbeing. Different stereotypies are likely to have different triggers, but studies have linked all of them to captive management, especially the feeding of low-fibre, high-energy diets and housing horses individually in stables with few opportunities for social contact. Stereotypies are a symptom of domestication and captivity.

Prevalence studies have found nearly a fifth of stabled horses display stereotypic behaviours. A popular explanation for stereotypical behaviour is that it is a sign of boredom, but there is little evidence to support this. Rather, in addition to dietary influences, it is more reliably explained in terms of behavioural frustration, as in other species. Horses, despite thousands of years of domestication, remain highly motivated to move about over open ground when they choose, search for food and have social contact with other horses. When these highly motivated behaviours are prevented by stabling, this internal motivation may find expression as stereotypic behaviour. Regardless of how well painted a stable block is, or how many hanging baskets of flowers increase its aesthetic appeal for humans, we should not forget that stables are horse 'cages' and that many horses spend significant proportions of their time caged.

Another popular belief is that horses can learn stereotypies by watching other horses and then copying them. Again, no scientific evidence supports this and a more reliable explanation is that when a second horse on a yard begins stereotyping it is because they are exposed to the same management practices as the first. The belief in copying can, in fact, be harmful when owners decide to isolate stereotypic horses so that they cannot be copied by others. Limiting opportunities for social contact in this highly social animal is linked to the development of stereotypies. So not only is such a measure ineffective, it may also exacerbate the problem and further diminish the wellbeing of the horse who is condemned to isolation.

As in other species, stereotypic behaviour is associated with a reduced quality of life for the animal performing it, but attempting to prevent the behaviour without addressing underlying causes can reduce quality of life further. Typing 'cribbing collar' into a search engine displays a selection of devices used to physically prevent crib-biting horses from performing their abnormal behaviour. Most comprise a leather strap which is tightened to the point that the horse can no longer flex their neck. Others incorporate a device for delivering a mild electric charge which is activated by the horse's neck action. Some owners arrange electric fencing around the inside of their horse's stable to punish crib biting, while others apply bitter-tasting substances. Some even have surgery performed on their horses to cut key muscles and nerves necessary for the behaviour. For weaving, anti-weaving bars may be applied to the stable door, to prevent the horse from swaying.

The effect in all cases of physical prevention, agreed by animal welfare researchers, is that the horses' distress is likely to be further increased. Owners may believe that preventing stereotypies is in their horse's best interests, linking the behaviour to various health problems. While it is true that stereotyping horses can struggle to maintain weight and may excessively wear their teeth down, claims that stereotypies are the cause of a variety of serious medical conditions are largely anecdotal. Therefore, the most humane and intelligent approach to stereotypical behaviour would be to prevent it from developing in the first place. Weaning practices are important in this regard, as is turn out to pasture. Unsurprisingly, steps that allow horses to behave as horses are found to be effective.

Gastric ulcers and stereotypies are not the only consequences for horses in a human world; chronic respiratory disease and colic are other important problems. For an animal adapted to life beneath miles of open sky, the enclosed space of a stable can have consequences for a horse's physical health. Airway disease can be a particular problem for stabled horses and is most commonly triggered by allergens such as dust and mould spores from feed and bedding. These inhaled particles are associated with the asthma-like conditions inflammatory airway disease and recurrent airway obstruction, which can afflict horses with a persistent cough and breathing difficulties. Inflammatory airway disease has been described as a disease 'primarily of domestication'.

Then there is colic, feared among horse owners and one of the most common causes of death in horses. I was very familiar with it, as Liverpool Veterinary School is globally a leading treatment and research centre for the condition, so I had already witnessed a number of the 350 colic cases that are seen at the hospital there every year.

Colic is the term used to describe the behavioural signs associated with abdominal pain. There are many different medical conditions which may cause this pain, including twisting of the gut and hernias. For mild pain, behavioural signs can include frequently turning to look at their flank and/or pawing at the ground. Horses in moderate pain may appear restless, repeatedly lying down and getting back up again. When in severe pain, horses will sweat, paw at the ground intensely and roll about violently.

The different causes of colic require different treatments and have different risk factors but some now-familiar risks are implicated. 'Sufficient access to pasture', for example, is proposed as important for reducing recurrent colic risk, while horses displaying crib biting, wind sucking or weaving have been found to be at increased risk of colic recurrence. In a scientific review paper on equine colic, published in *The Veterinary Journal*, Professors Chris Proudman and Debbie Archer also note that an increased number of hours spent stabled can increase risk. They concluded:

> Given that the equine gastrointestinal tract evolved to cope with trickle-feeding it is perhaps not surprising to discover the role that current management practices play.

It is hopefully apparent from the foregoing that these problems afflicting horses are not the result of deliberate cruelty, but rather a widespread mismatch between a horse's evolved biological nature and their ability to exercise that nature in our human environments. This discrepancy does not have sufficient physical and functional impacts to prevent equine industries from thriving (horses can still be competitively ridden, for example), in the same way that barren battery cages do not stop hens from laying eggs. But its psychological impacts have significant effects on the quality of horses' lives which, at present, society may frequently be blind to.

Of the millions of people who watch the equestrian disciplines at the Olympics, for example, few probably think about the horses' quality of life beyond the showing arena. This is not intended to detract in any way from the determination and excellence displayed by the riders, nor to pass judgement on the fans, but my remit is to consider the horses' experiences when their doting trainers, riders, grooms, chiropractors, massage therapists and others are stripped away.

A glimpse into these horses' lives beyond their minutes of performance is gained during the BBC video 'Horses dance to Phil Collins in Olympics dressage', from the 2012 Olympics, where the commentator reveals that the performing horse 'had a minor blip with some colic surgery a couple of years ago'. That the horse is back 'competing' at the highest level is a tribute to the veterinary surgeons who alleviated substantial suffering and no doubt saved the horse's life. The same horse defecates in front of the adoring crowd as the commentator delivers her line, as though relieved that public acknowledgement of his digestive health has been forthcoming. The 'performance' – the sequence of movements the horse has been trained to make – is simply another period in time when he must try to fulfil his physical and psychological needs as a horse within the human world in which he must cope.

Animal welfare researchers Professor John Bradshaw and Dr Rachel Casey found that 81 per cent of horse owners thought that their animals could feel 'pride'. Pride is a complex emotion, requiring self-awareness, and there is no unequivocal evidence that it exists in dogs or even chimpanzees, let alone horses. One risk of this anthropomorphism is that we do not consider the animals' species-specific needs. Another is that these assumptions about mental capabilities might sometimes result in punishment, because owners think that their animals have knowingly and wilfully done wrong. I remember being behind the scenes at a horse show in the UK, where a frustrated rider returned from a round in the ring that had clearly not gone the way she intended. She angrily blamed the horse, smacking him on his head and neck, and forcefully yanking down on his bridle with each furious question posed. 'Why did you ignore X? Why didn't you do Y? Why were you so lazy after all our hard work and training?' She may have simply been venting her anger or, if one of the 81 per cent, she may have been struggling to comprehend her horse's perceived loss of pride at such a critical moment.

Dressage horses are undoubtedly lavished with high levels of individual attention, but are noted for having demanding training regimes and extensive periods of individual stabling. In a survey of management and training practices for UK dressage horses, the majority of the horses were stabled for 64–91 per cent of their time, whether competing at elite or non-elite levels. This can be because space for turn-out to pasture is at a premium and because owners are concerned that the horses will injure themselves if left to their own devices in a paddock, especially if turned out with other horses. The perceived magnitude of such risk, however, may not be well supported by research or veterinary experience. Leading equine veterinarian Dr Midge Leitch, for example, noted that stable-confined horses are more likely to sustain training injuries and have high levels of pent-up energy from inadequate opportunities to stretch and relax.

In addition to the substantial percentage of dressage horses who would be expected to have stomach ulcers, a separate survey found that a third were reported to display abnormal behaviours, a finding which was correlated with their time spent stabled. Similar to the result we saw for dairy cows, horses have also been found to become more optimistic when they are given access to pasture and other horses, after being kept singly in stables.

Other familiar and high-profile uses of horses include pleasure riding and racing. Just under a third of horses and ponies in Great Britain are reported to be overweight or obese, with pleasure horses being more than twice as likely to be obese compared to competition horses. Horses with obesity have not only a reduced quality of life but also an increased risk of laminitis (painful inflammation within the hoof) – a fact which has prompted awareness-raising obesity campaigns from the British Equine Veterinary Association and charities such as the UK-based World Horse Welfare.

Racing is familiar to most as a result of nationally famous events, such as the UK's Grand National, run less than ten miles from my childhood home nearly every year since 1839. The National is described as the most famous steeplechase in the world, attracting an estimated worldwide viewing audience of 500 million people. Clearly, its epic four-mile course and thirty demanding jumps prove to be an exhilarating and unpredictable spectacle for observers, many of whom have little or no interest in horse-racing at any other time of the year. But it is widely known, and apparently increasingly covered in the media, that to create such a spectacle and to retain its unpredictability, there must be an element of risk to both the horses and riders. Sixty-six horses are reported to have died at the Grand National Meeting (a three-day event, including the Grand National race) and the high-profile Cheltenham Festival in the ten years to 2019. According to the British Horseracing Authority, in the five years to 2020, 848 horses died on racecourses in British racing.

Dr Mark Kennedy, senior scientific manager for equines at the UK's RSPCA, points out that these deaths are not 'freak accidents', but predictable. The risk of horse fatalities in British jump racing is around 4 per 1,000 starts, while the figure for flat racing, without jumps, is lower at around 1 per 1,000 starts. Comparing this to the risk of driving a car once a day, Dr Kennedy notes that if there was the same degree of risk as for horses in jump racing, a driver would be lucky to still be alive after nine months. He comments, 'I doubt many car drivers would accept this level of risk.'

In response, trainers and race course officials frequently point out that no sport can be risk-free, with a spokesperson for Aintree Racecourse suggesting that the Grand National is a 'tough but fair test for horses'. A top trainer also drew a comparison between horseracing and driving, pointing out that, no matter how safe major roads are made, there will always be accidents. Such a response, however, assumes that horseracing and driving are both essential activities, which can only, at best, be made as safe as possible. Few would argue that major roads should be closed to fully eliminate driver risk, but some would question whether horseracing for human entertainment is as necessary as key transport infrastructure. There also remains a question as to whether horses would want to be 'tested' (with risk of serious injury and death), if given the choice. Some commentators note that risk of injury is an integral aspect of sporting endeavour for both human and equine athletes. But the ability to choose whether to compete, and expose oneself to that risk, remains a critical ethical distinction between the two.

Another aspect of horseracing that feeds into society's moral judgement has been the use of the whip by jockeys, particularly when a whip is used to 'encourage' a horse to run faster, and the public's acceptance of whipping an animal in the name of sport. There have been changes to whip-use rules in recent years, and developments such as the introduction of a more humane whip with a cushioned, shock-absorbing design. But headlines around whip use continue to appear.

Media coverage of fatalities and whip use, rather than just the sporting triumphs of the races themselves, may be indicative of a shifting social ethic. There was angry public reaction following the 2011 Grand National, when a BBC commentator euphemistically referred to the two horses lying dead on the racecourse as 'obstacles' that the remaining running horses were required to bypass. A decade later, in 2021, a leading Irish trainer made headlines, and received a 12-month ban, for being photographed sitting and apparently posing on a dead racehorse who had died during training.

In 2022, a survey by the Equine Ethics and Wellbeing Commission of the International Federation for Equestrian Sports found that the majority of the public, 67 per cent, in 14 countries think that horses do not enjoy being involved in sport or only enjoy it sometimes. The Commission's international survey of the equestrian community – those working with horses – also found that the majority, 78 per cent, believe that animal welfare standards need improving.

When assessing overall welfare costs to animals, whether the animals are being used for sport, food or any other human purpose, it is important to consider the various sources of possible welfare compromise, in addition to those in the public eye. For horses, social contact and companionship from other horses, the ability to move freely in open space (through turn-out to pasture) and access to roughage such as grass, hay and/or straw are especially important. Restrictions of these basic needs must be identified and accounted for, alongside race fatalities, whip use and other high-profile issues such as the treatment of former racehorses – as featured in the 2021 BBC *Panorama* documentary, 'The Dark Side of Horse Racing'.

We have already seen that the majority of racehorses in training have gastric ulcers and that up to a fifth of stabled horses exhibit stereotypical behaviour. With these points in mind, it is pertinent to examine claims that, whatever risks racing may present for horses, their indulgent care off the course affords racehorses a good life. The former jockey Richard Pitman, for example stated:

> I've been with horses all my life and I've never seen a horse that hasn't lived really well. I have seen and looked after so many and I can say I'm happy they have had a good life.

It is also frequently asserted that horses enjoy racing. Pitman, for example, said, 'Horses are bred to race and in the National, when they fall, they can't wait to get up and carry on.'

It is certainly true that horses are herd animals. Like many prey animals, their evolved predator-avoidance response is one of fight or flight. So as soon as one horse responds to danger, perceived or real, all of the horses in a group will react, galloping together away from the threat. Recalling that the behavioural responses of domestic horses have changed little during domestication, this group fleeing, coupled with their training, is likely to be what we are seeing when rider-less horses continue to run and jump. The observable flight reaction alone does not reveal how some rider-less horses are feeling as they continue to gallop and jump, though in light of its evolutionary origins the behaviour may be as likely to be motivated by fear as pleasure.

It is difficult to see beyond the crowded stadia, cheering crowds and the billions of pounds of bets placed each year. Though many who enjoy equestrian activities may not have explicitly considered it, the accepted ethical justification is that humans *enjoy* using horses for sport and leisure; they enjoy getting dressed up for a day at the races and having a flutter (a British term for placing a bet), or watching a horse and rider execute meticulously rehearsed manoeuvres in an arena. Utilitarianism is the ethical theory that weighs costs against benefits and guides the 'right' course of action based on maximizing overall happiness. There is no doubt that equestrian activities generate human happiness, both for participants and spectators, but this must be weighed against the list of welfare compromises to the horses.

If the current body of evidence suggests that competition and captive management results in significant negative welfare impacts for horses, and if ethical analysis concluded that such impacts cannot be justified by human enjoyment (which can be achieved by numerous alternative means), what prospect is there that a culturally significant event such as the Grand National would eventually be run for the last time?

Such a question is being asked in Australia. New South Wales, where Australia's first jumps event was held in 1832, banned jumps racing in 1997 under the state's Prevention of Cruelty to Animals Act 1979 and every Australian state has stopped jumps racing except Victoria. It is true that the Grand National is an established tradition in the UK, but tradition is used to justify a variety of sporting uses of animals which many British citizens may find unpalatable. These include Spanish-style bullfighting and Washington's Suicide Race. In the latter competition, horses are raced down the steep 69-metre Suicide Hill towards the Okanogan River, which they must cross and then sprint towards a waiting crowd in a rodeo arena. Twenty-five horses are reported to have died taking part in the race in the 36 years to 2018 (compared to twenty-six in the same period in the Grand National). The Suicide Race is an 86-year-old tradition, said to provide a significant economic boost to the host town of Omak.

Britain's equine industry also has a significant economic impact, with horseracing reporting, in 2020, 5.77 million attendances at 1,500 fixtures, an annual expenditure of over £3.5 billion and a tax contribution of over £300 million. Yet some of the most morally objectionable activities in human history were defended on the grounds of economic importance, serving as a reminder that economic contribution does not necessarily make an activity morally justifiable.

For many years during my childhood, the blue riband hare coursing event, the Waterloo Cup, was staged in the nearby fields of the Altcar Withens, as it had been annually since 1836. During the three-day event, wild hares were beaten from nearby cover out onto a field, where greyhounds were set free to chase them. The dogs were judged on their ability to turn in response to the hares' agile escape attempts, cheering onlookers betted on the outcome, and a percentage of the hares were caught and killed. Each year the local media, in response, would contain a rash of reports about protests at the Waterloo Cup and debate about its acceptability in a civilized society. The event historically drew tens-of-thousands-strong crowds and in the late 1860s its three-times winner, greyhound Master McGrath, was said to be a household name in Britain.

I looked in from the boundary fence of the Waterloo Cup once and remember a racecourse-like atmosphere, with lots of excited betting and alcohol. I don't really remember whether I ever believed it would end, but in 2004, with the passing of the UK's Hunting Act, it did. Interestingly, the Waterloo Cup was inaugurated by Liverpool's William Lynn, who also organized the first Grand National.

The role of horses has shifted enormously throughout human history, having been variously instrumental for war, transport and agriculture. Now, in the developed world, horses are used mainly for leisure and entertainment. Their continued use in sport is funded and maintained by our betting and viewing. The industry is taking steps to change. In 2020, the racing industry's Horse Welfare Board published a strategy for the welfare of racehorses. Charities such as World Horse Welfare are actively promoting the Three Fs for horses – freedom, friendship and forage – championing cultural change to ensure their regular turn-out to pasture, opportunities for social contact and constant access to high-fibre food. In 2019, these same recommendations were included in the EU Animal Welfare Platform's good practice guide to horse keeping. In 2022, the Pony Club Australia focused their new horse welfare policy on the horses' positive mental experiences, rather than simply their physical health. Some leading racehorse trainers, such as Venetia Williams and Rebecca Curtis in the UK, are promoting the benefits of turn out to pasture and companionship to horses. On the Happy Horses section of her website, Curtis says 'They are horses and herd animals at the end of the day and it's probably quite boring for them to be stuck in their boxes 23 hours a day when they're not ridden, so ours go out and have a roll, and it keeps them eating and healthy.'

It is not a given that the current usages of horses by humans will endure. The lives we allow domesticated horses to lead are decided by us and this must surely be guided by our ethics and influenced by our increasing understanding of their experiences. For their sakes, we should continually question the acceptability of their roles, our direct and indirect participation in them, and the social licence upon which all equine activities are based.

Throughout my visit to California, there had been the prospect that, at the end, I could join a boat trip out across the vast submarine canyon within Monterey Bay. Plunging for a mile, the Monterey Canyon is one of the deepest in the US, comparable in size and shape to the Grand Canyon. It is relatively close to the Californian shoreline, offering visitors and researchers exceptional opportunities to witness the rich marine life, including great whales, which its size and depth can support.

I stood at the back of the boat facing seaward and scrutinized the visible open water up to the point where it merged with an encircling foggy boundary. Specks of salty mist pricking my lips and cheeks found fleeting connections with a bristling sense of possibility.

'OK!' The American accent burst through the speakers. 'We gotta *blue whale* at five o'clock!'

My heart began banging in my chest. I gripped the rail and looked out behind the gently bobbing boat. Suddenly, midway towards the impenetrable fog, a rushing plume of spray ejected skyward. It was the sound that was unexpected: the gushing exhalation of a giant – the largest known animal to have ever lived – above the muffled breeze. A watery sequoia thundered up above the whale, nourished by tons of centimetre-long krill, and melted into the mist.

Next came the whale's bluish-grey back, an almighty hulk of flesh rolling through the water's surface. From the perspective of the boat, nearly level with the whale, it was impossible to appreciate the enormity of the animal beneath, but the permanence of their dorsal surface transiting through the hazy air left little doubt. It kept coming: more and more of the great mass leaving and entering the water like a magician's handkerchief. In the scale and grinding progress, I sensed the shifting of tectonic plates that had gouged the whale's canyon home into the face of the Earth. And in the few minutes that they could be observed moving through the water, the blue whale effortlessly assimilated all of my thoughts and experiences from my weeks in California. As I focussed intently on nothing more than the colossal creature's moving back, they casually absorbed my observations and concerns. I was momentarily freed as each left my mind and attached like barnacles to the whale's body as they arched their back more prominently and threw their fluke, one of the most enigmatic sights in the whole of the natural world, high up into the sunlight, to the coos and exclamations of the watching audience. The sun gleamed off the whale's wet skin and reflected through the waterfalls now pouring from the tail fin as the whale dived for a final time.

CHAPTER 11

Our animal companions

I drove home from my final exam staring at the flicking wiper blades brushing pouring rain from my windscreen, convinced of my failure. I couldn't remember any of the questions but knew that some of my answers were, frankly, ridiculous.

Results day followed, with its disaster movie scenes of hugging, crying and consoling. I walked past smiling representatives of a local business who had sponsored jam scones, and joined the emotional fray to look at the results board. Then I removed myself, walked across the grounds of the veterinary field station where I had spent two years following families of swallows, nuthatches, jays and little owls, and stutteringly revealed to my parents on the telephone that, somehow, I had fulfilled my lifelong ambition of becoming a veterinary surgeon.

I was offered a job at a veterinary practice in the north-west of England and began work early in January with a 'small animal and exotic' caseload. I was to start earning a living tending the animals that people keep as pets, or companion animals, including some of the more unfamiliar varieties, such as reptiles and various birds.

The ability of veterinary surgeons to serve the interests of animals through euthanasia when their quality of life is judged to be intolerably and unimprovably poor is well known, and such consultations, emotionally demanding for the vet and owner alike, soon became a part of my everyday life.

Euthanasia is often a time of great sadness and the occasion that most openly reveals the depth of attachment that people can have for their pets. For some, the animal is a last remaining link to a deceased spouse, and older owners in particular tell fond tales of how their pet and former husband or wife used to live their lives in close, affectionate partnership. For others, their pet has clearly become a source of strength and invaluable companionship following the death of a spouse, an observation verified by studies. In one study, among recently widowed women, pet owners were found to be emotionally and physically more resilient to the stressful effects of bereavement.

Perhaps most revealing for me working in a practice seeing exotic animals was the variety of species to which people became attached. It seems that any pet's loss is keenly felt when they have become part of the family routine and have made their carers felt needed. A well-built man in a high-visibility jacket came to the practice during a break from a local building site, explaining that he was concerned about a lump on his family's pet rat. I examined the inquisitive creature and had to break the sad news that this was almost certainly a tumour. The man did not want to opt for diagnostic tests or possible surgery and he placed his two hands palms-down on my consulting table and began to shudder from his shoulders. As I, and all veterinary surgeons, have become accustomed to, he began to tearfully recount what life with his small friend was like: the animal's preferences, her ability to make his children laugh and how she would curl up on a lap or tuck herself into a shirt pocket if the family sat down to watch television. He clearly demonstrated how much he cared for his animal and the hole that would be left in the family's everyday experience when she was no longer with them.

Emeritus Professor of Animal Welfare at the University of Pennsylvania, James Serpell, notes that some people (typically not pet keepers), as well as expressing surprise, dismiss or denigrate such human–animal relationships as strange or ridiculous. But as Serpell points out, pet keeping is such a widespread human phenomenon, through history and between cultures, that it must serve some meaningful purpose to those who practise it. For the world's millions of pet keepers – including those who may be economically disadvantaged and yet still opt to take on an animal who must have their care needs paid for – a substantial body of evidence suggests that they are deriving valuable benefits of companionship, pleasure and, in some cases, emotional support.

By working at the coalface of these human–animal relationships, veterinary surgeons, as well as becoming aware of how much pets mean to people, also become aware of how such relationships impact upon the animals themselves. The strength of attachment may become a source of conflict if, for example, a highly bonded owner is unwilling to euthanize an animal who is clearly suffering with an untreatable condition. In these cases it is incumbent on the veterinary professional to proceed sensitively while maintaining a sharp focus on the animal's best interests. For vets, like most people, it is apparent that the principle of fairness demands that, for the benefits that companion animals bring to us, we should, in return, give them the things that they need to be healthy and happy. Working as a general veterinary practitioner offers some insight into whether pet owners are meeting their side of this ethical bargain.

Early life experiences have a significant impact on an animal's future temperament and wellbeing. Three processes are particularly relevant – socialization, habituation and training.

Anyone who has reared puppies or kittens will be aware that in their first few weeks of life they are highly inquisitive, approaching and exploring anything new. At this time, their brain is soaking up these experiences like a sponge, creating a reference bank that they will draw on throughout life. This is known as the socialization period and is a time when anyone with responsibility for rearing companion animals must carefully expose them to a variety of other animals and people – men, women, old, young, people wearing hats, people in wheelchairs, people from different ethnic backgrounds and so on. Doing this carefully means that the breeder or new owner should watch for signs of fear, as a fearful interaction could create a lasting aversion rather than a positive association. Similarly, the process of habituation involves carefully exposing young animals to everyday sights and sounds, such as dishwashers, vacuum cleaners and washing machines. Again, the young animals should first hear these sounds at a distance and then gradually more closely over ensuing days.

In puppies, between the ages of approximately three and fourteen weeks is particularly important for ensuring adequate socialization and habituation, while in kittens the first seven weeks of life are considered most influential. This means there is a particular onus on those who breed pet animals to ensure they provide a suitable living environment throughout pregnancy and up until the animals are transferred to their first owners. This, together with a variety of positive experiences continuing when the young pet is at their first home, gives the animals the best chance of becoming friendly, outgoing, well-adjusted family pets.

Many of the problem behaviours that develop in pets can be traced back to inadequate socialization and habituation. Dog owners, for example, will sometimes report that their dog 'doesn't like men' and may suspect past mistreatment. While a previous bad experience with a man *can* cause future fear and aggression towards men, failure to be socialized towards men during the socialization period can also, and more commonly, have the same effect.

Puppy farms – where puppies are bred on a large scale, with little regard for their, or their parents', welfare – may not only be dirty and disease ridden, but also result in puppies who spend their socialization period in barren, unstimulating pens and are then sold to become family pets in an urban environment that can become a source of lifelong fear and anxiety. This longstanding problem became particularly acute during the Covid-19 pandemic, with concerns that unscrupulous breeders cashed in on the high demand for so-called 'pandemic puppies'.

Hearing recordings of fireworks and similar noises during the socialization period – starting off quietly and gradually getting louder – can protect dogs against firework fears and phobias, which affect around 40 per cent of all dogs in the UK, or 3.8 million dogs. Gradually accustoming young puppies to being left alone is the most effective prevention against separation-related behaviour – the distressing howling, barking, pacing, house destruction and/or indoor toileting displayed by an estimated fifth of pet dogs in the UK, 1.9 million, who struggle to cope when left alone by their owners. The PDSA Animal Wellbeing Report, the UK's largest annual assessment of pet wellbeing, reports that a fifth of pet dogs in the UK are left alone for five hours or more on a typical weekday. This figure, unsurprisingly, nearly halved during Covid-19 lockdowns, but had been unchanged in the ten years to 2020.

Poorly socialized animals are among those most likely to be relinquished with behavioural problems to rehoming centres, or sadly to be euthanized for problem behaviour, such as aggression, when all other options have been explored. Between 2015 and 2018, 23,078 people were admitted to UK National Health Service hospitals for dog-related injuries, and over a fifth of whom were children and young people. Researchers at the UK's Royal Veterinary College found that a third of deaths in dogs aged under three years (roughly 21,000 deaths annually in the UK) are caused by problem behaviours, with euthanasia accounting for most of these deaths. As well as a sad loss of life, this places a significant emotional toll on veterinary surgeons and nurses.

The third important behavioural process, training, involves deliberately teaching animals rather than simply exposing them to sights and sounds.

It was probably during a visit to France, aged around 12, when I first became aware of the significance of training companion animals. Two things struck me during a daily visit to a local farm. First, that some of the farmer's dogs were treated affectionately as pets, living indoors, while others were considered as working animals and kept permanently chained outside until needed for their jobs. This seemed unfair. Second, that if the dogs gave unwanted attention they were told to 'Allez!' That is, they were all (unsurprisingly in hindsight) spoken to in French. It made me wonder whether they understood French. And if they did, do other dogs understand German, Hungarian and so on? This seemed strange to my young mind, because, if so, who had taught them?

An important way in which dogs learn is by associating certain words and gestures with things that consistently follow them. So if removing a lead from a hook in the house always results in being taken for an enjoyable walk, then it may not be long before even reaching for the lead can send a dog into a frenzy of excitable spinning and barking. The dog's owners may even need to speak of the 'L-E-A-D', knowing that saying the word in full will send their dog into the same joyous lather.

When hearing a spoken sentence, a dog may recognize their frequently-used name (which may have little significance to them, besides getting their attention), but unless any of the other words in the sentence have been consistently paired with a particular outcome over time, they may all be meaningless. Dogs who are told off by their owners may learn an unpleasant association with their owners' threatening body language and tone. But how are our companion animals to understand the myriad rules of human society, if we do not take the trouble to teach them?

Professor John Bradshaw describes the common occurrence of owners shouting at their dogs when they fail to return to them: a scene that I am familiar with at the more human-visited parts of Formby Beach. It begins with a dog being freed from their lead, into an endless space where they can run in circles, chase gulls and investigate children playing football until they are exhausted. The problem comes when the owner is ready to leave before their dog has had enough of this unbounded pleasure and calls the dog's name, expecting them to obediently return. Frequently, however, the dog has never been trained to understand this recall signal, or not in such a stimulating environment, the owner simply expecting that their dog will understand the words. So the running continues, tongue lolling gleefully, and the owner becomes increasingly irritated and embarrassed. They start shouting more angrily ('I've had it! Understand?...'), and when the dog finally returns on their own terms, some owners shamelessly administer what they see as justifiable physical punishment.

From the dog's perspective, two things have happened. First, by only ever being called when it is time to go home – and never for anything enjoyable, for training purposes – the dog has learned that returning leads to their enjoyment ending (of course, it can't be explained to them *why* their fun can't last for ever). Second, to compound this, they have learned that when they do return, or at least sometimes, they get hit, angrily shouted at and/or viciously shaken by the collar. So, for the dog, there is nothing to motivate them to return, or there is a fear of doing so, which leads to further 'disobedience' (in the owner's eyes) and a vicious cycle of punishment and non-returning. As John Bradshaw observes, 'It is more logical and straightforward to train dogs to come back to their owners because they want to.'

A related issue is overlooking that pet animals are constantly being inadvertently trained through our interactions with them. Every time an owner gives their pet attention, for example by stroking them or feeding them a treat, they are effectively communicating, 'Well done, I am giving you something nice for what you are doing now.' An owner may give titbits from the dining table, but then, on a future occasion, tell their dog off for pestering or begging. They may give warmth and affection when their cat joins them on their bed at the weekend, but reject them during the week. The world can be a confusing place for companion animals, particularly if such inconsistently applied rules are coupled with unpredictable verbal or physical punishment.

Finally, when owners *do* seek to train their dogs, some of them are still attracted to methods that seek to challenge a dog's perceived dominance. Animals can be humanely trained to repeat desirable behaviours through the administration of carefully timed rewards until a request is learned, through a process called positive reinforcement. This is humane, and animals learn more effectively because they are in a relaxed, positive emotional state. Dominance-based training theory demands that owners exert physical superiority to ensure that their dog cannot ascend above them in a supposed all-important social hierarchy. Despite such an approach being promoted by some high-profile celebrity dog trainers, there is nothing to support the commonly held view that an owner must be seen as the pack leader in their dog's eyes. Practices such as an owner ensuring they eat before their dog or pinning their dog to the ground to 'show them who's boss' are, at best, meaningless and, at worst, inhumane.

An important aspect of consultation skills taught at university was to first determine an animal's signalment – their age, sex and breed. An older cat's increased thirst may be more likely to indicate kidney failure, a female dog's vomiting might be linked to an infected womb and so on. But the breed was also instructive when creating lists of possible diagnoses. A coughing Cavalier King Charles Spaniel could signify heart disease, while itching and scratching in a West Highland White Terrier raises suspicion of allergic skin disease. The reason is that, once again, selective breeding of animals by humans for desirable traits has unintentionally selected for undesirable traits that affect the animals' health and wellbeing. In the case of dogs, animals were originally selected for breeding if they showed certain useful behavioural tendencies, such as a propensity to guard territory or herd livestock. Then, more recently (over roughly the last hundred years), they were increasingly bred for having certain appealing appearances. This has not just been the case for dogs; Persian cats have been selected to have a flat face, Munchkin cats to have short legs, Bubble-Eye goldfish to have large fluid-filled sacs projecting from beneath their eyes, fancy pigeons to have feathers covering their eyes, corn snakes to have unusually coloured scales and so on. Professor James Serpell suggests that some physical traits, such as the wrinkles around the eyes and drooping jowls of certain dog breeds, may have been unconsciously selected to produce permanent facial expressions which 'evoke human sympathy and indulgence'. But whatever the underlying reason, it is now known that many health and behaviour problems have arisen from selective breeding and, whenever these are identified, continuing to breed, regardless, results in knowingly prioritizing aesthetic appeal over the animals' quality of life.

The health problems may be of two main types. First, by selecting for a physical trait (such as a flattened face), the genes for an inherited disease may also be accidentally selected for. Persian cats have a characteristically flattened face, but around a third are also susceptible to developing polycystic kidney disease – a disease in which multiple fluid-filled kidney cysts gradually enlarge until kidney failure results.

The second type of problem is linked to the animal's shape and physical characteristics themselves. Breeds including English Bulldogs, French Bulldogs and pugs, like Persian cats, also have a flattened face and all of these breeds (including the cats) are affected by brachycephalic obstructive airway syndrome (BOAS). 'Brachycephalic' means shortened head, which results because the upper jaw and nose of the skull are greatly shortened. The soft tissues inside the nose and throat, however, are unchanged, so must squeeze into a smaller space. They become narrowed, making it more difficult for air to flow through them and this is why brachycephalic dogs can often be heard snoring and snorting as they try to breathe normally. The bulldog, often called the British Bulldog, is frequently depicted in association with the Union flag and identified as a symbol of British cultural identity. But the reality for many bulldogs and other brachycephalic breeds is that they are unable to breathe freely and experience problems such as recurring skin infections and eye ulcers, and are typically unable to give birth without requiring a Caesarian section. Many will undergo surgery to correct abnormalities, such as narrowed nostrils, an overly long soft palate or a narrowed windpipe. On their Genetic Welfare Problems website, the Universities Federation for Animal Welfare (UFAW) explains that BOAS in bulldogs causes 'Snoring, respiratory noise, mouth breathing, respiratory distress with rapid breathing and struggling for breath, and can lead to collapse and death. Dogs with BOAS are unable to take even moderate amounts of exercise, are very prone to heat stroke and have constantly disrupted sleep.' The British Bulldog may evoke patriotic notions of spirit and determination but this and other brachycephalic breeds, which have soared in popularity in recent years, symbolizes nothing positive about the United Kingdom's historic attitude towards animal breeding and wellbeing.

The UK's Brachycephalic Working Group, composed of charities, academics, breed health representatives, the UK Kennel Club and veterinary associations working together to improve the welfare of these dogs, has a simple and unified public message: 'Stop and think before buying a flat-faced dog.' The group also supports the appropriate use of legislation. Animal welfare laws applying in England since 2018, and Scotland since 2021, state that a dog may not be kept for breeding if 'breeding from it could have a detrimental effect on its health or welfare or the health or welfare of its offspring'. To date, there has not been a test case.

In a Royal Veterinary College study of owners whose dogs were affected by BOAS, over half reported that their dog did not have a 'breathing problem', despite their pet showing frequent, severe clinical signs of the condition. Dr Rowena Packer and her co-authors cautioned that a perception of such signs as 'normal' in brachycephalic dogs could hinder efforts to improve the problem through altering breeding programmes.

Owner misperceptions have similarly been associated with another common health problem affecting companion animals – obesity. Over half of cat owners with an overweight cat, for example, believe that their cat's shape is as it should be. Pet nutrition has advanced in recent decades, such that most dog and cat owners now feed complete commercial diets – complete meaning that they contain appropriate nutrients in the correct amounts. However, many owners may regularly overestimate how much of this food their pet requires and, additionally, some 6 million pet dogs, cats and rabbits in the UK are regularly fed treats, including chips, cheese and cake. In consequence, around four out of every ten pets who came through my surgery door were classed as overweight or obese. I would break the sad news that loved pets had developed diabetes linked to their weight and would require daily insulin injections; prescribe anti-inflammatory medication to manage the painful arthritis of hobbling dogs; recommend surgery for ruptured cruciate ligaments in overburdened knees; and try to sympathetically convey to owners how their pet's breathlessness, reluctance to exercise and unwillingness to play were all signs of their reduced quality of life due to permanently carrying excessive weight. Nevertheless, in owner surveys just under half report that feeding treats 'makes my pet feel happy', while over a quarter report that it makes them (the owner) feel happy. There can be a disconnect between the satisfaction of seeing a pet's delight at being offered treats compared to the misery of the same animal being diagnosed with a serious weight-related medical condition or dying two years prematurely. Overfeeding and obesity give clear examples of the relationships that must be considered between mental wellbeing and physical health when considering an animal's overall welfare. There were moments of gladness, however, when, following weight clinics with our veterinary nurses (offered by many veterinary practices), owners would report how happy they were to see their dog or cat's renewed vitality and how nice it was to 'have their old pet back' – who, in many cases, had gradually deteriorated as the weight had crept on over several months, without the loving owner realizing.

A common problem for cats is chronic (longer-lasting) stress and this was sometimes revealed at the practice through cats who were presented for having blood in their urine and/or difficulty urinating. Such signs were the result of frequent exposure to stressors in the cats' home environments, which are associated with changes to the protective layer in a cat's bladder. Stressors for cats in modern households can include things like building work (such as a new kitchen), a new baby, a new pet or the presence of other unrelated cats. Adult cats show variable degrees of sociability and many prefer not to live with other cats. They may choose to interact with other cats, especially those they have grown up with as littermates, but they value having that choice and being able to seek privacy when they want it. In the UK, around four and a half million cats live in a household with another cat, with some owners opting to acquire a second cat as a 'friend' for their existing cat. Owners may not see overt aggression between their cats, but may not be aware of subtle behavioural signs, such as intentional avoidance, lowering their ears when walking past each other or one cat sitting in certain locations to block access to another. That said, the owners of over two million UK cats do perceive such signs, reporting that their cat lives with one or more cats whom they don't get on with.

In multicat households (if these cannot be avoided) the key to minimizing chronic stress is to ensure all of the cats have individual access to the facilities they need, such as litter trays, feeding bowls, resting and hiding places, and so on. A general rule of thumb is to provide one of each of these items for each cat, plus one spare (for example, three litter trays for two cats), and to space them out around the house, even if the cats have outdoor access. In the UK, just 4 per cent of households with two cats provide three or more litter trays and half provide one or no water bowls, increasing the risk of chronic stress and painful urinary tract disease.

Rabbits, the UK's third most common mammalian pet, were frequently admitted for treatment of advanced dental disease. This involved opening their small mouths as wide as possible under general anaesthesia and using a powered dental burr to file down chisel-sharp spikes on their teeth. Rabbits, like horses, have evolved to spend 70 per cent of their time above ground grazing, but it became the norm to feed them high-carbohydrate, low-fibre diets which are harmful to their digestive and dental health and do not meet their psychological need to graze and forage. If rabbits were fed at least their own body size in good quality hay every day, with opportunities to graze on growing grass whenever possible, a handful of suitable fresh greens such as broccoli and cabbage twice daily, and just a tablespoon of grass-based shop-bought rabbit nuggets, many of the dental problems we were required to treat could have been prevented. But with a constantly filled bowl of traditional rabbit muesli – a mix of seeds and flakes – and with insufficient hay, a rabbit's constantly growing teeth are not worn down. In consequence, their front teeth may grow out of their mouth and curl round to penetrate their facial skin; their back teeth may develop sharp spurs, which cause sores and ulceration on the tongue or inner surfaces of the cheeks; and the tooth roots commonly elongate to compress structures such as the tear ducts or even, in some cases, grow backwards into the eye socket.

Today, a fifth of the UK's pet rabbits are fed insufficient hay. While this equates to 189,000 rabbits still not receiving enough dietary fibre, this figure has halved in the last 10 years and the percentage feeding muesli-type food has dropped from a half to a fifth in the same period. This is likely thanks to concerted education and awareness-raising from charities, veterinary associations and some pet food manufacturers.

Any rabbit owner planning to transition their pets to a more suitable diet should do so gradually, slowly introducing nutritious food and phasing out muesli mixes over the course of around two to four weeks, to avoid a dangerous digestive upset caused by sudden dietary change.

One owner presented a rabbit to me in a carrier, then separately handed me the animal's tail in a matchbox. She had been keeping two unneutered male rabbits together and escalating aggression had finally caused the tail injury. Several rabbits were also brought to me with injuries to their scrotum, with a similar story. Some could be immediately sutured, others required treatment for infections.

Like other domesticated animals, rabbits retain many of the behavioural motivations and social preferences of their wild ancestors. Anyone who has noticed rabbits grazing on grassy road verges will recognize their tendency to forage in pairs or groups; rabbits naturally live in family groups of 2 to 14 members, in an underground warren that may house over 100 individuals. In a study of domesticated rabbits using consumer demand methodology (as mentioned in Chapter 2, the scientific approach of asking animals how much they value certain provisions), animal welfare scientist Dr Shirley Seaman added increasing weights to doors through which rabbits could access various resources. With rising entry costs (increasing weights), the rabbits reduced their number of visits and stayed for longer, demonstrating that the extra effort was affecting their choices. But Seaman and her colleagues found that the rabbits' motivation to gain contact with another rabbit through wire mesh came close to their motivation for accessing food, suggesting that they value this highly. Despite their strong preference for companionship, many pet rabbits are kept individually, with 48 per cent currently living alone in the UK. This, however, is down from 67 per cent living alone in 2011. There are 432,000 pet rabbits still experiencing social isolation, but initiatives such as the UK veterinary profession's #ItTakesTwo campaign are seemingly having an impact. It is important, however, that a rabbit's companion is one they can get along with, or aggression and injuries will result. If rabbits are to be kept as pets, without unwanted breeding and fighting, a neutered male with a neutered female is a recommended combination.

As for cats and dogs, certain behaviours can become problematic for the owners of other species, despite being appropriate for the animals.

One lunchtime, the practice receptionist came running upstairs into the staff room and said that one of us had to come to see a man at reception immediately.

'Ee's dead angry!' she said in her Liverpudlian accent. 'Ee's sayin' he wants a parrot killed!'

Each of us looked at the others around the table and I volunteered to go down.

I arrived at the front desk to find a man in his forties, wearing a black leather jacket, pacing.

'Would you like to come through?' I asked with an upbeat tone. The man spun round to face me.

'Listen mate, I don't wanna discuss anythin' with ya, all right? I just want the parrot killed. I don't wanna talk about it, I just wannit over, shall I go and get the bird now?'

I tried to gauge the man's body language.

'Do you want to just step inside for a moment,' I said, gesturing towards the consulting room. He walked in and resumed pacing.

'What's been happening?' I asked carefully, closing the door. The man was flushed in his cheeks and seemed on the verge of tears.

'Look mate, I'm at the end of me tether with the bird. I don't wanna talk about it… It's the only thing… I've made me mind up, OK? D'you want me to go and get it now? I've got a taxi running on a meter outside mate, so I don't wanna talk t'you about it, all right?'

The owner was clearly distressed but I could not simply act as a pet disposal service and had a duty to the bird to explore possible solutions.

Problem behaviour is not uncommon in pet parrots and I wondered if this could be the issue.

'OK. I'm not going to be able to take an animal from you without asking you a few questions and asking you to sign a form,' I said with a slightly firmer tone. 'I just need to ask you what kind of bird it is and what's been happening.'

'The taxi's on a meter, mate... She's a cockatoo... She's cracking, I've had her for years, but I've got a new girlfriend and the bird hates her. She's always screaming and bites her... so I want 'er killed, all right?' He paused. 'I can't go on like this.'

It seemed that the man was very attached to his pet cockatoo but was trying to distance himself from the emotional reality of his difficult decision.

'OK. Is she just aggressive towards your girlfriend?'

'Yeah, she's a cracker with everyone else. But she screams if I'm with my girlfriend and tries to attack her if she goes near. She said she's going to leave me if I don't get rid of the parrot.'

'Could anyone else give her a home?' I asked.

'No, mate, no one wants her, this is the best thing.'

'OK, do you want to bring her in?'

He walked out to the waiting taxi and returned with a cage. Inside was a beautiful white cockatoo with dark inquisitive eyes and a bright yellow crest. She was in pristine condition with perfect, sleek feathering. It was clear that I was not going to be able to persuade the man to seek behavioural therapy and I feared for the bird's safety if she was returned home. Our practice worked with a local charity that could care for unwanted parrots.

'Would you be happy to sign her over to us and we'll find a home for her?' I asked.

The man looked at me. 'I don't know, mate.'

'Or you can get good results with someone who specializes in pet behaviour problems.'

'No chance, mate, if I take her home alive me girlfriend'll leave me.' I looked at him. 'If you can find a good home for her, I'll sign the form.'

The sulphur-crested cockatoo spent a week at the practice in a large room which we converted into an indoor aviary, before a space became free with the charity. She was tame and mild-natured, sitting on my hand and offering the top of her head to be scratched whenever I went in to sit with her.

I first encountered wild, free-living parrots in Uganda. They were difficult to spot in a canopy of tall trees, but were in a large flock that maintained contact with piercing, far-carrying squawks. Their physical and social environments were complex and varied, and once in a while small numbers of the birds would take to the sky, flying high and fast overhead into the distance. Wild parrots regularly fly several miles between feeding sites and typically spend between four and six hours each day searching for, selecting and manipulating different food items.

Pet parrots, in contrast, are often housed alone in a cage and may be occupied by their bowl of readily available food for less than an hour each day. This leaves them with much time to be filled. The vast majority brought to see me were also being fed unsuitable diets. Their owners were buying bags of sunflower seeds labelled and sold as parrot food resulting, like rabbit owners, in them unwittingly malnourishing their pets.

Many parrots were also brought to the practice with a highly visible problem. Bald across their whole body, besides the parts they could not reach such as the head, they would spend time each day chewing and removing their own feathers. This so-called feather plucking has been estimated to affect 10 to 15 per cent of all captive parrots. It is a complex condition to treat, with a variety of possible triggers. As well as medical causes, such as underlying pain or skin irritation, other triggers include a dry, centrally heated living environment without opportunities to bathe or be sprayed, and wing clipping, where owners cut their parrot's flight feathers to prevent flight. Aside from its contribution to the development of feather plucking, many veterinary and behavioural experts are opposed to wing clipping, as parrots are eminently trainable, renowned for possessing cognitive abilities comparable to toddlers and can be taught to return on command. As specialist veterinary surgeon Dr John Chitty has written, 'If owners wish to have a non-flying pet, they would be well advised not to get a bird.'

As for my beleaguered cockatoo, insight into the possible explanation for her behaviour is provided by researchers at the University of Bern. Dr Rachel Schmid and her colleagues examined the common practice of removing captive-bred parrot chicks from their parents to be reared by humans, known as hand-rearing. If parrots are to be kept as pets there are important benefits to breeding them in captivity rather than trapping them in the wild, but elements of a parrot's normal behavioural development depend on early contact with their parents. When this is denied and substituted with human contact, the birds become highly adapted to being handled by people and are often sold as 'cuddly tame'. Such parrots seem particularly affectionate and suited to life as pets until, as young adults, they may select a specific human being as a partner. At this stage, they may begin screaming when separated from their human partner, as they would to regain contact with a partner in the wild, and begin aggressively biting anyone who approaches the object of their affections. Unfortunately for the bird, their owner cannot satisfy their social requirements and the resulting behavioural frustration leads to intolerable tensions such as those suffered by my client, his cockatoo and his girlfriend. As with problem behaviours discussed for dogs, while treatable with the help of an accredited pet behaviourist, this is a common reason for relinquishment and requests for euthanasia of otherwise healthy animals.

After one and a half happy years working in Liverpool, I moved to Somerset in the south-west of England to work as a veterinary locum. Each region of the British Isles has its own wildlife jewels and I was soon to experience species that I had not previously encountered in the north.

I arrived at Shapwick Heath early on a May morning, joining a long, straight path that bisected the 500-hectare national nature reserve. The sprawling landscape had a mellow simplicity: endless reedbeds glowing yellow beneath the rising sun, blue sky dressed with white spiderweb clouds and the mystical Glastonbury Tor rising through a misty backdrop beyond. I was in the heart of the Somerset Levels enveloped by the frantic chattering of warblers newly arrived from Africa.

As the day warmed, freshly emerged dragonflies filled the sky with iridescent specks of food. Then one by one, also recently arrived from tropical Africa, small, colourful falcons came to hunt them, carving through the open vista upon sweeping parabolic trajectories. Commonly hailed as the only bird fast and agile enough to catch a flying swift, the hobby resembles its relative the peregrine, but is smaller, with striking red feathering at the tops of its legs and a swept-back curvature to its wings. There were as many as 30 ahead of me, slicing through the sky's harvest in 6,000-year-old echoes of the Neolithic sickles that once hacked the landscape beneath. Their powering, purposeful arcs terminated with precise last-moment adjustments to snatch their insect prey, followed by a momentary glide as each morsel was dexterously transferred from their talons to their hooked beak. Then a resumed burst of acceleration propelled them fast and high, leaving a confetti of discarded wings fluttering in their wake.

As well as a rich variety of wildlife, including, in winter, millions-strong murmurations of starlings, Shapwick Heath is home to the Sweet Track, the second oldest timber trackway discovered in the British Isles. Constructed around 4,000 BC, large parts still exist, preserved by the reserve's wet peat. As I walked among the reeds, I mused on our long associations with companion animals.

Throughout history, pet keeping has been popular among the world's ruling classes, but in 18th- and 19th-century England the practice spread downwards from the aristocracy. Professor James Serpell links this trend to the decline of anthropocentrism – a human-centred world view – and the gradual development of a more equal approach to animals and the natural world. Over half of all households in the UK now own at least one pet and it is through sharing our homes and lives with these animals that we are able to appreciate their individual habits, preferences and personalities: qualities which form the basis for empathy, prompt us to acknowledge the resemblance of companion animals to ourselves and to attribute animals with sentience. Some studies suggest that this may lead to more sympathetic attitudes towards animals more generally.

But as the status of companion animals has been raised towards regarding them as members of the family, there is a risk that we treat them as people. Dogs can be bought 'puppuccinos' in cafes. When the idea spread to include 'puguccinos' for pugs, veterinarians cautioned against offering sweetened whipped cream to a breed whose breathing difficulties are exacerbated by obesity. In 2017, the British Veterinary Association's Senior Vice-President, Dr Gudrun Ravetz, said that pug-themed cafés are 'all about the human owners, rather than the health of the pet'. Meanwhile, the global pet clothing market is reported to have grown 8 per cent in 2020, projected to reach 7 billion US dollars in 2028. Dressing pets in clothes they don't need, feeding them human foods such as chips and cakes until they develop obesity, or acquiring a cat as a 'friend' for an existing cat who would prefer to be alone are examples where affection and good intentions are not aligned with good animal wellbeing. The PDSA Animal Wellbeing (PAW) Report, documenting and quantifying issues outlined in this chapter, has concluded that many of the UK's pets are:

'Stressed. Lonely. Overweight. Bored. Aggressive. Misunderstood [...] but loved.'

In Ancient Greece, some of Pythagoras' thoughts on animals were recorded in *The Teachings of Pythagoras*, including:

Have done with nets and traps and snares and springes,
Bird-lime and forest-beaters, lines and fish-hooks.
Kill, if you must, the beasts that do you harm,
But, even so, let killing be enough.

Over 2,000 years later, these words rang true as I was given an opportunity to contribute to a debate on the future of the trade in wild-caught birds imported into the European Union to be kept as pets.

The UK's Animal Welfare Foundation invited me to give a talk on parrot welfare at their annual discussion forum in London. Normally, this would have covered topics that I've outlined, such as the malnutrition, lack of stimulation, feather plucking and screaming affecting a proportion of the UK's pet parrots, but the timing of the talk had an additional topical relevance. A case of H5N1 avian influenza – a disease threat to domestic poultry and potentially people – had been detected at an avian quarantine facility in Essex, UK, where imported wild-caught parrots and other birds were being held before onward distribution as pets. In consequence, a temporary ban had been placed on the importation of wild-caught birds in to the European Union, something that animal welfare and conservation groups had been lobbying for since the early 1990s. The current situation gave an opportunity to highlight the trade's harmful effects.

First, the risk of importing dangerous pathogens had been demonstrated by the case of avian influenza. This ever-present risk from increasing human encroachment on wildlife populations has risen to global prominence in the Covid-19 pandemic. Second, the parrot family faces a higher rate of extinction than any other comparable bird group, with habitat loss and the pet trade identified as principal sources of endangerment. Third are the animal welfare implications occurring at each stage of the supply chain. Capture methods, to this day, include the bird lime that troubled Pythagoras – a gluey substance applied to branches where birds are known to perch, sticking to their feathers and preventing them from flying away. Alternatively, tethered call birds may be used to attract other birds, allowing spring-loaded nets to capture an assembled flock. The birds are handled and packed densely into crates by the trappers and passed to dealers who travel between villages, collecting birds for sale to exporters. Trappers, dealers and exporters may all pack large numbers of birds tightly together in cages at holding facilities, where there is little or no knowledge, resources or regard for minimum care standards. Poor conditions lead to pre-export mortality rates of 40 to 66 per cent, arising from poor handling, inadequate provision of food and water, hyperthermia, inadequate ventilation, infectious disease outbreaks and aggression. More birds then die during international transport and quarantine, with UK government figures of between 1 and 12 per cent. Before arriving at pet shops to be sold, approximately six in every ten wild-caught birds will have died.

I concluded my talk by quoting a letter from a veterinary surgeon who was responsible for an avian quarantine facility, published in the *Veterinary Times* two months earlier:

When the crates were opened, many of these birds were dead or moribund and others were severely distressed. They were then put into quarantine. The suffering of these birds from shock, transport, crating, change of climate, dehydration, etc. I found unacceptable. Whereas the trade has been stopped to control the spread of disease,

I think that the cruelty aspect of the trade is as important, if not more so. Even when they were released from quarantine, the suffering did not end. Sure, some went to well-run aviaries, but many were incarcerated in cages in private dwellings to satisfy the whims of the owners.

For a profession concerned with animal welfare, disease control and the protection of global biodiversity, there was a clear relevance to my veterinary audience.

Debate ensued, exploring the necessity of the trade and possible implications of a permanent ban. While it was true that local people derived income from trapping birds, much of the profit flowed to intermediaries. Additionally, the trade denied local communities the opportunity to derive long-term benefits from their native wildlife as the harvest was unsustainable – many species were being trapped faster than they could breed. Perhaps most importantly, the trade was unnecessary as many of the birds that people wish to keep as pets can be bred in captivity in the European Union. This must be done knowledgeably and humanely, and does not automatically solve the other welfare problems currently associated with captive husbandry, but it prevents the suffering associated with capture and long-distance transport.

Two months later, the British Veterinary Association (BVA) President, Dr Freda Scott-Park, announced that the veterinary profession was calling for the current ban on the import of wild birds to be made permanent because of concerns for the welfare of the birds during capture and transit.

Further action followed swiftly. The BVA statement was adopted by the Federation of Veterinarians of Europe, becoming the stated position of the veterinary profession in Europe, who lobbied as part of a coalition including the Royal Society for the Protection of Birds (RSPB) and the World Parrot Trust. A week later the British Prime Minister wrote to the coalition partners to relay that the UK government was to press 'for the present temporary ban on wild birds being imported into the EU to be extended indefinitely'.

I joined our coalition partners to present the veterinary view at the European Parliament and Commission and was soon experiencing similar gut-wrenching feelings of nervousness and hope that had preceded my veterinary finals. I arrived early for my final meeting at the European Parliament building in Brussels and decided to take a stroll in the local parkland. It was the first week of December, and as the various facts continued to circulate around my mind ahead of the meeting, a shrill call penetrated the cold air from the trees above. I looked up and could see a pair of birds moving acrobatically through the upper branches. They looked roughly thrush-sized with a long tail and a heavy-looking bill; one of them repeated their call. It was not a call I was familiar with among parkland birds, but it had a squawking quality that transported me back to Uganda and my consulting room in Liverpool. Then one swooped down to a nearby bush, revealing their unmistakeable identity. Emerald green with a red beak and a pink and black collar – a ring-necked parakeet. Clambering among the leafless branches, the parakeet, quickly joined by their partner, gave a vivid and unexpected reminder of the brilliance, sociability and wide-roaming habits of the animal whose relatives we were advocating to protect around the world. I was aware of feral populations of these birds in various European cities, including London, but had no idea that Brussels was one of them. As the sun began to set, I gained a final glance of the birds, silhouetted against the soaring parliamentary towers behind, and resolved to make my small contribution – articulating the veterinary profession's views as clearly as I possibly could – one last time.

The future of the EU wild bird trade remained a preoccupation over Christmas, then news came on 11 January 2007 that a permanent ban on the importation of wild-caught birds into the European Union had been agreed. A month later, the magazine of the World Parrot Trust carried the front page headline 'Fly free... forever!' beneath a photograph of a free-flying blue-fronted amazon parrot, celebrating legislation that would spare around four million wild birds every year.

A year passed quickly, with another surge of birds crossing the planet in harmony with the Earth's endless orbiting around the sun. I drove to a remote Forestry Commission car park in the Somerset countryside on a July evening, with the possibility of seeing another beguiling African migrant, here to raise their youngsters on a summer of flying insects.

The sun had dipped below a large pine plantation when I arrived, leaving the air feeling cool on my face as I set off through the woods, jumping over exposed tree roots with bracken brushing against my legs. The track opened onto a more substantial path flanked with looming dark conifers, which began winding up a hill. Behind me, the headlights and distant hum of occasional cars passed along the country road, but as I reached the top only my quickened breath and the dusk chorus of a song thrush disturbed the still air. Ahead, the mature plantation gave way to an area of shorter, younger trees, in rows before the orange sky.

I stood still, listening to the thrush's repeating exclamations as the sun shrunk along its reddening avenues. The hilltop fell silent and I sat down on a fallen log, still listening.

After a few minutes, a soothing, slightly mechanical churring sound began emanating from within the young trees. It continued in long phrases, sending its rippling vibrations through the forested plateau and around me like an invisible masseur. The churring stopped and there was a high-pitched yelp. I strained my eyes to see if I could make out the shape of any creatures perched on top of the trees, but nothing. In the distance, red lights shimmered along the length of a tall telecommunications mast and the otherworldly churring resumed.

Suddenly the silhouette of a bird with outstretched wings appeared above the path, flapping hectically and jinking from left to right as though being pulled by kite strings. The light was dim, but bright enough to make out a white flash on each of the bird's wings. It flew close as though keen to inspect me. I held my breath as the bird moved even closer and I stood, for a few magical moments, beneath the beating wings of a hovering nightjar.

With large eyes and a huge gape, the slim, blackbird-sized nightjar lies motionless and camouflaged on the ground throughout the day, emerging at dusk to hunt large moths. Being nocturnal and with their repertoire of strange sounds, including the slowly rising and falling churring song which can be heard throughout the night, these birds have long engaged the curiosity of those who encountered them. Some say Aristotle was the first to mention the mistaken belief that nightjars sucked milk from goats and other livestock at night, giving rise to their scientific name, *Caprimulgus* – the milker of goats.

The nightjar dipped across the path and disappeared above the trees opposite, sounding a sharp crack as they clapped their wings together. I sat back down on the mossy log and reflected on the parrots, and the animals that I was seeing and treating during my working days.

The animals we have welcomed into our homes as pets have become loved family members. But love is a feeling in our minds and can only be appreciated by animals through our actions towards them. Being loved has no positive meaning for an animal if it is not translated into actions that promote their health and wellbeing.

The Five Welfare Needs enshrined in the UK's Animal Welfare Acts were introduced in Chapter 1. UK pet owners have a legal obligation to meet these five needs, but meeting them is also the translation of an owner's love that is meaningful from the animal's perspective. The late philosopher Professor Bernard Rollin described the legislation as Britain's 'quality of life law'.

For animals to enjoy their lives as human companions, human knowledge, attitudes and care-giving practices need to further evolve. In some countries, animal sentience is still barely recognized. In others, such as the UK, many animals have become the objects of our great affection. It is good for animals that we recognize their preferences, personalities and similarities to us when we keep them as companions, but that is not the same as anthropomorphically assuming they are the same as us. Critical, or rational, anthropomorphism recognizes the important similarities, but also recognizes that animals have species-specific needs which are different to our own and are increasingly understood.

As UK citizens understand that legal duties accompany car ownership and motoring, so awareness of the Animal Welfare Acts and their Five Welfare Needs should grow so that the similar responsibilities that now accompany pet ownership are understood. Veterinary associations and animal welfare charities are working hard to make this happen.

Pre-purchase advice and the sourcing of animals to create demand for those who are healthy and well adjusted are critical. A growing percentage of prospective pet owners are visiting their local veterinary practice for advice – veterinary professionals are very keen to provide this information, are not too busy to do so (as some people fear) and the pre-purchase consultation is typically offered for free or low-cost.

The Animal Welfare Foundation and RSPCA have developed a legal puppy contract for prospective puppy buyers, together with an accompanying puppy information pack. Freely downloadable at www.puppycontract.org.uk, it seeks to guide owners before parting with often large sums of money, to ensure that the puppies have been socialized and habituated, and the parents tested (where applicable) for heritable diseases before breeding. The breeder then signs the contract to verify this. A similar kitten checklist, launched in 2019 by the Cat Group – a coalition of the UK's leading veterinary and animal welfare organizations dedicated to feline welfare – is freely available from the Cat Group website. If prospective pet owners were only to buy healthy, happy pets, only healthy, happy pets would be bred. Currently, according to the PAW Report, nearly a quarter of UK pet dog, cat and rabbit owners said they did no research before acquiring their pet.

For puppy buying, the purchaser is advised to see the puppies interacting with their mother in their rearing environment; if this happened, dirty, barren puppy farms, devoid of opportunities for socialization and habituation, would become a thing of the past. In April 2020, Lucy's Law came into force, meaning that anyone wanting to get a new puppy or kitten in England (with similar legislation in Wales and

Scotland) must now buy direct from a breeder, or consider adopting from a rescue centre. Licensed dog breeders are required to show puppies interacting with their mothers in their place of birth.

If all pet owners were aware of the Five Welfare Needs – environment, diet, behaviour, companionship, health – and met them, the routine, preventable problems that contributed to my daily veterinary caseload would fade away. Rabbits would be housed in accommodation that allowed them space and resources for exercise and exploration, and cats would not become stressed through insufficient provision of key resources such as litter trays (environment). Rabbits would be fed predominantly hay instead of rabbit muesli, parrots would not subsist on nutritionally inadequate sunflower seeds and all pets would be spared the excesses of frequent unhealthy food treats (diet). Young pets would be socialized, habituated and trained using kind and effective methods, and owners would recognize that problem behaviours always have an underlying motivation that can be addressed with professional assistance (behaviour). Highly social animals like dogs and rabbits would not be left alone for long periods, nor would cats be required to live with other unrelated cats they don't get on with, leaving them susceptible to chronic stress (companionship). All animals would be bred with regard for their health and future wellbeing – avoiding harmful shapes and sizes, and utilizing widely available tests for genetic diseases (health).

In addition to knowing how to meet these Five Welfare Needs, prospective owners also need to have the means to be able to do so. In recognition of this, the national UK veterinary charity PDSA structures advice on a prospective owner's lifestyle and circumstances around the acronym 'PETS', prompting them to consider:

- **P**lace – how suitable for a pet is the place where you live?
- **E**xercise – how much exercise could you give your pet?
- **T**ime – how much time could you spend with your pet?
- **S**pend – could you afford the monthly expense of your preferred pet?

We have grown to love the animals we keep as companions and recognize the richness of their characters, but we continue to maintain a psychological separation from many of the farmed animals who also provide us with great benefits, are similarly characterful, but live their lives distant from the comfort of our homes. We directly influence the lives of our companion animals through the care and resources that we provide for them, but we pay someone else to provide the same for the animals who enter our homes as food. For as long as we lavish our pets, aside from whether our love results in them leading good lives, yet continue to buy food with little regard for the animals that yielded it, there will continue to be the paradox well described by Professor James Serpell:

> At one extreme are the animals we call pets [...] We nurture and care for them like our own kith and kin, and display outrage and disgust when they are subjected to ill-treatment. At the other, we have animals like the pig [...] supremely useful animals in every respect [...] and in return for this outstanding contribution, we treat pigs like worthless objects, devoid of feelings and sensations [...] The quality of life we impose upon them suggests nothing but contempt and hatred.

Perhaps as we learn more about the pleasures and pains of animals, and

257

continue to be reminded of their interests through the close daily contact we have with our pets, we can now extend five-needs-based care to *all* the animals whose quality of life we fund, both directly and indirectly: the dog lying beneath the table and the chicken being carved on a plate above. Millions of pets and millions of farmed animals would benefit from our extra attention and efforts in these areas. Though the scale of the issues can seem large, the case of the EU wild bird trade demonstrated to me that with a sound case, commitment and collaboration with others, animals' lives can be changed for the better.

CHAPTER 12

The power of one

There is a simple pleasure in strolling with a well-worn pair of binoculars and following changing seasons and landscapes through wild sights and sounds. I drove into the Somerset countryside an hour before sunrise, past frozen fields and glassy dykes. Eventually reaching a muddy lay-by at the entrance to a lakeside copse, I stepped out of the car and breathed furls of vapour into the morning air as I pulled on a final few warm layers. A small gate opened onto a footpath and I entered the wood at first light.

Once in the enclosed copse my senses, as always, ignited picking forensically through every rustle and disturbance. Subconsciously, I began side-stepping crinkled leaves and fallen branches that might draw attention. My eyes scanned through the leafless branches, working together with my straining ears to locate the source of every slightest sound. Any thoughts more complex than those giving rise to a bristling, sensory exploration of the wood and its inhabitants were excluded.

I saw movement in my peripheral vision and spun my head, locking onto a small patch of foliage. Another blur of movement and a small brown wren alighted on a moss-covered rock, pivoting jerkily from left to right beneath their tiny cocked tail. I continued my cautious progress along the earthen track, further into the wood.

Next there was a splash, triggering my sensitized mind. The white undertail of a moorhen disappeared along an overgrown ditch, the bird puncturing the cold air with a sharp characteristic yelp.

Then came the pinprick calls of a tiny bird in the canopy ahead, causing me to stop dead in my tracks and re-focus my tightly grasped binoculars with renewed concentration. This time, it was the smallest bird in the UK, the goldcrest, affording fleeting views as they flitted high above me. I was close. But there had been recent sightings here of a similarly beautiful bird that I had never seen before.

The path ended at a wooden barred fence, leading onto a private farm track. The sun had risen and, with little cloud cover, the wood was brightening through the leafless trees. I sat on the fence and rubbed my gloved hands together.

Away from human habitation, my thoughts turned to the variety of opportunities that exist to gain similar contact with the natural world, from the simplicity of a back garden or local wood to an organized excursion in a far-flung land. I was conscious that such opportunities are declining as the world becomes ever more crowded and wondered how civilizations might persuade themselves of the value of such opportunities, in order that they might be preserved.

For anyone who has not seen the world's human population graph, it is like a rocket's trajectory, ascending near vertically. It is relatively level in the 18th century, begins visibly rising in the 19th century and blasts off dramatically in the 20th and 21st centuries. Every species on the planet, whether a bacterium, a birch tree, a goldcrest or a whale, goes through a similar rapidly rising phase in their population size, but then something becomes a limiting factor – they may run out of space, food, or an infectious disease might become established because of the higher density of individuals – and the rate of population growth begins to slow. It is worth remembering that an oak tree may produce hundreds of acorns, and breeding pairs of blue tits may lay ten or more eggs during each of their reproductive years, but the numbers of oak trees and blue tits in the world are not rising indefinitely. When the population of a certain kind of plant or animal reaches a more or less steady level, the population is said to be at the carrying capacity of the environment for that particular species.

The pattern for humans, however, is slightly different. We have evolved a brain that is particularly effective at problem-solving – our so-called intelligence – and this has allowed us to overcome many of the typical population-limiting factors. We have, for example, developed agriculture so that food is in constant plentiful supply, materials to make homes and clothes to protect us from the elements, and medicine to treat many of the diseases that would otherwise kill us at younger ages. In consequence, many humans are capable of breeding and surviving, and this is reflected in our ever-growing global population.

Superficially, this sounds highly successful, but it presents humans with different problems. Our numbers are growing, but our only home is a planet with finite space and resources. This puts us in competition with all the other species on the planet who rely on the same limited resources as us. The winners of this competition – usually humans – continue to survive and breed, while the losers eventually die out. Accordingly, the planet is now inhabited by a highly dominant and influential species – us.

The Earth's four-and-a-half-billion-year history is divided by scientists into various distinct periods, including the familiar dinosaur-inhabited Jurassic period. To reflect the substantial impact of humans on the planet, the current geological period is referred to as the Anthropocene – the period in which humans have become 'the architects of their own planetary future'. This period is characterized by a million animal and plant species heading towards extinction as humans exert various influences, from deforestation to grow crops, to harvesting wildlife faster than it is able to replenish. Around one in seven of the world's bird species, for example, are threatened with extinction.

The Anthropocene has also seen a warming of the climate, mostly attributed to a rise in carbon dioxide, methane and nitrous oxide – greenhouse gases – which have increased since the onset of the Industrial Revolution. Climate change is causing rising average temperatures, sea level rises, acidification of the oceans and more intense storms and sea surges, making the world a more challenging and inhospitable place in which to live.

The Earth may be considered to have a natural carrying capacity for humans, as for all species, but our problem-solving brains may permit us to exceed it. The One Planet Living initiative points out that if everyone in the world lived like an average European or North American, we would need three or five planets, respectively, to live on. The exact figures are debated, but it is clear that consumption of natural resources per person varies widely between countries and the highest consumption levels could not be sustained or expanded while keeping humanity within safe environmental limits, or 'planetary boundaries'. As the United Nations says, 'Economic and social progress over the last century has been accompanied by environmental degradation that is endangering the very systems on which our future development – indeed, our very survival – depends.'

It is also our brain, however, that is allowing us to identify the problems associated with exceeding the Earth's carrying capacity. Our scientific method has allowed us to measure and monitor declining populations of species, for example, as well as study conscious awareness and indicators of wellbeing in a wide range of animals.

In a world of ruthless competition between all species where the fittest survive, humans could turn a blind eye to such discoveries and continue proliferating unchecked. But in addition to intelligence, we have evolved morality – a sense of what is right and wrong, justifiable and unjustifiable – and our impacts on other species have led to conservation concern and concern for animal welfare.

It seems, then, that with a science-guided awareness and moral concern about our impacts, we ought to be interested not only in how we could flourish across the planet, but how we should. Flourishing has connotations of prosperity as well as expansion. Our species may be clever, but do we live up to our scientific name of *Homo sapiens* – 'wise man'?

The concept of sustainable development attempts to capture such thinking and is being pursued by governments around the world working towards the United Nations' Sustainable Development Goals. Sustainable development is sometimes described as being able to do tomorrow what we do today, but there are great problems in the world, including poverty, inequity, malnourishment and lack of clean drinking water, so sustainable development is about more than just carrying on. Environmental philosopher Dr Kate Rawles has noted that sustainable development is therefore ethically aspirational.

Sustainable development has traditionally been constructed around three pillars – environmental, economic and social – with development in each area resulting in an overall direction of progress recognized as sustainable. A difficulty with this traditional model is that it does not obviously capture the wellbeing of the billions of sentient animals with whom we share the planet, although their humane treatment should be considered a hallmark of social progress and development. The UK government's advisory Farm Animal Welfare Committee (now Animal Welfare Committee) advocates the three Es of environment, economy and ethics, in which animal welfare is central to public acceptability and therefore ethical sustainability. Either way, bolstered by the findings of animal welfare science, animal welfare must urgently be afforded the high priority it requires.

Interest and concern for the natural world and the wellbeing of animals are interwoven. Early morning walks in wakening woodlands offer opportunities to stop and reflect in a busy world. Careful observation may reveal rare and secretive creatures and moments to the wildlife watcher, whose fascination and delight lead to a greater commitment to their protection. The same careful animal observation is how animal welfare scientists have been able to validate certain animal behaviours as indicators of underlying feelings, such as the subtle tail flicking of lambs, castrated and tail-docked without anaesthesia or analgesia. These findings, when disseminated, lead to greater commitment to develop and support ethically sustainable husbandry practices. It is recognized that the physical health and productivity of farmed animals can give some indication of the animals' welfare, but that these measures alone give an incomplete assessment. Having additional regard for the evolutionary history of kept animals, which logically flows from knowledge of the natural world, and insisting on opportunities for them to express elements of their normal behaviour that they value is not to argue that an animal's captive husbandry should be informed by a romantic notion of nature. Instead, it recognizes that domestication is a minor evolutionary event in geological time and that domesticated animals retain behavioural motivations that arose during their evolutionary past – the thwarting of which can lead to frustration and suffering, and the permitting of which can lead to pleasure. Similarly, the Biophilia Hypothesis, proposed by the late Harvard Professor Edward O. Wilson, posits that humans have an evolved tendency to affiliate with nature and wildlife, which if thwarted harms our emotional wellbeing. Time spent in nature, for example, offers a space for reflection and psychological restoration, as I have relied on all my life and as so many have rediscovered during Covid-19 lockdowns. According to Wilson's collaborator, Professor Stephen Kellert, conserving nature may represent less an ethical act of kindness than 'an expression of profound self-interest and biological imperative'.

It is evident to large numbers of people that the extinctions, loss of natural spaces, changing climate and institutionalized harms to animal wellbeing are having practical and emotional consequences for humans. These features of the Anthropocene are detectable locally. When certain houses in my childhood town of Formby have been demolished in recent years and rebuilt, developers have decided that any future owner would no longer want hedges or grassed lawns. Beech hedges that as a child I had repeatedly visited, excitedly reaching up on my toes to sneak careful glimpses of nesting song thrushes and blackbirds, were torn out as a priority. These same birds, like many others, relied on the grassed lawns for finding food such as earthworms. Nationally, nearly a quarter of UK front gardens have been paved over – a tripling in a decade – to provide space for car parking, reducing wildlife habitat and contributing to local flooding.

How, then, can more people be persuaded to consider such impacts? Human self-interest is a powerful motivator, and benefits need to be demonstrated. Recall that a ban on the EU wild bird trade attracted convincing animal welfare and conservation arguments, but that it was the demonstrated risk of importing infectious disease, with capacity to infect humans and have an economic impact on the domestic poultry industry, that ultimately sealed its fate.

Interest and enjoyment in seeing wildlife, and relaxation provided by greenery, may be expressions of Wilson's Biophilia Hypothesis. There is strong and consistent evidence for mental health and wellbeing benefits arising from exposure to natural environments, which is now influencing government health policy. Numerous studies have revealed psychological benefits including reductions in stress, fatigue, anxiety and depression. Additionally, these benefits increase with the amount of biodiversity – grassland, woodland, plants, butterflies, birds and so on – in a given area of public greenspace. Spaces with higher biodiversity, that are well maintained (for example, being kept free from litter) and in which people feel safe, are those most closely associated with improved health.

Recognizing these benefits of contact with the natural world for human health and wellbeing, it is concerning that the proportion of children in high-income countries playing outside in natural spaces has dropped significantly compared to previous generations. Time spent interacting with electronic devices has risen over the same period, prompting research into the psychological impacts for children and adolescents of screen time versus green time. A report commissioned by the National Trust, Europe's largest conservation organization, focussed on a proposed nature deficit disorder affecting Britain's children, characterized by physical health problems including obesity, mental health problems and a declining ability of children to assess risk to themselves and others.

In 2020, the UK government launched its first ever People and Nature Survey for England, aiming to provide ongoing official statistics to understand the role of nature in the nation's health and wellbeing – an indicator in itself of the priority now being afforded to this area. In the inaugural survey, against the backdrop of the Covid-19 pandemic, 87 per cent of adults agreed that 'being in nature makes me happy'. Among children aged 8–15, 83 per cent agreed that being in nature made them very happy, rising to 94 per cent of children who reported spending time outside noticing nature and wildlife. The coronavirus lockdowns have, however, highlighted inequalities in access to nature and green spaces, with public health professionals cautioning that disadvantaged communities have significantly less access – not only to their own gardens or other outside space, but also to green space within 300 metres of their home. Of children from ethnic minority backgrounds or from households with an annual income below £17,000, 71 per cent had reported spending less time outside since coronavirus, compared with 57 per cent of white children or from households with an annual income above £17,000. Encouragingly, environmental concern was high among children across all socioeconomic groups, with 78 per cent saying that protecting the environment was important to them.

The benefits that resources and processes in the natural environment provide to humankind are known as ecosystem services. Opportunities for reflection and inspiration are themselves forms of cultural ecosystem services, alongside supporting services (such as essential nutrient cycling), provisioning services (such as food, water, energy and medicines) and regulating services (including absorbing carbon dioxide from the atmosphere). Salt marshes and coastal wetlands may be places of hauntingly beautiful wilderness, but in his book *What Has Nature Ever Done For Us?* Tony Juniper describes how intact coastal wetlands protected the south coast of the US from Hurricane Rita in 2005, three weeks after the similarly intense Hurricane Katrina had killed more than 1,600 people in New Orleans. Notably, the New Orleans' coastal marshes had been cut to create shipping channels, compromising their ability to reduce the height and energy of the storm surge.

Analysed in this way, benefits of protecting the natural world are clear, but when governments and businesses are driven by financial gain – when economics predominates over environment or ethics – then somehow we allow these benefits to be sidelined and trumped. It seems critical that arguments in favour of protecting the living environment must always include the aesthetic, emotional, cultural, inspirational and spiritual, but recent years have also seen moves to value the natural world in explicit monetary terms. If money talks, then, so the reasoning goes, nature advocacy needs to incorporate the language of economics.

In 2006, Sir Nicholas Stern, commissioned by the UK government, concluded that benefits from spending money to reduce carbon emissions would far outweigh the costs of not acting, and increased political attention followed. Five years later, the UK's National Ecosystem

Assessment offered a similar economic analysis for ecosystem services with media headlines announcing the conclusion of 500 experts, that nature is 'worth billions' to the UK.

These economic approaches should help the natural environment compete as governments strive to boost struggling economies and recover from the Covid-19 pandemic, but the risks of neglecting inspirational value and intrinsic worth or overemphasizing economically justified conclusions are evident. As the Native American prophecy goes, 'When the last tree is cut down, the last fish eaten, and the last stream poisoned, you will realize that you cannot eat money.'

There are also economic benefits to improving the welfare of many kept animals, but in the case of farmed animals we have seen how profitability can be sustained despite poor animal welfare. For example, over a quarter of a commercially viable broiler flock may be painfully lame, or behaviourally restricted laying hens in battery cages will continue to produce eggs. As agricultural economist Professor John McInerney describes, there is a non-linear relationship between animal welfare and productivity. As humans begin to use animals, welfare initially rises as the animals benefit from provision of food and shelter, healthcare and protection from predators. But as productivity rises, due for example to increasing confinement and genetic selection for faster growth, the welfare of the animals begins to decline.

At this point, ethics must come to the fore so that, as a society, we can decide what amount of harm to our kept animals, if any, is justified. Where abject cruelty and malicious treatment is concerned, Chapter 10 highlighted the risks of such treatment becoming generalized towards vulnerable members of human society. This gives one reason for not tolerating such treatment towards animals. To increasing numbers of people, however, it is simply the capacity of animals to experience good or bad wellbeing that is most relevant. People recognize that when animals become dependent on humans for meeting their needs, a moral duty arises to treat those animals well. If a wild songbird is captured and placed in a cage, aside from the rights and wrongs of the act, most people realize that the bird becomes completely dependent on their captor for essential provisions. Most would view it as wrong to forget about the bird, let them go hungry and starve. They would not be similarly concerned about the wellbeing of an attractive rock or seashell collected on a walk; the bird's sentience is the moral difference.

A well-publicized example of our collective sense of moral duty towards sentient animals impacted by humans occurs when languishing seabirds are washed up on beaches following oil spills. In some countries there is widespread public support for attempting to clean the birds, spurred by a sense that humans should undo the harm that other humans have caused. The same people, however, do not usually advocate that humans should seek out injured or ailing seabirds at times other than oil spills. They do not feel that we are morally obliged to intervene with the animal suffering that is an ever-present part of nature, only that for which we are responsible, whether after an oil spill or on farms, in racing stables or in our homes.

Animal welfare science has provided evidence that an animal's needs go beyond simply providing what is necessary for survival, such as food and water, and beyond the basic requirement to avoid abject cruelty. They include other needs and opportunities that contribute to wellbeing and pleasure: for example, appropriate companionship, comfort, being able to express important aspects of their normal behaviour and to find interest in their living environments. To be able to thrive, as well as survive. Our sense of moral duty to meet the needs of captive or managed animals therefore extends to these needs as well.

In 2015, astronomers reported the discovery of Kepler-442b – an Earth-like planet in the habitable zone around a parent star not unlike our own. Extraterrestrial intelligence is yet to be discovered anywhere, but I would not be the first to point out that if a newly emergent intelligent lifeform ever decided that captive humans would provide them with many practical benefits, we would hope that our alien captors would take the trouble to understand and meet our needs for good health and wellbeing.

It has become apparent that all of the foregoing issues – the climate and biodiversity emergencies, and the health and wellbeing of animals and humans – are inextricably linked. The global human population is projected to peak at nine to eleven billion people around 2100, from its current level of just under eight billion. For organizations such as Population Matters, a UK-based non-governmental organization (NGO), limiting this rise through voluntary means – such as empowering women and providing universal, modern family planning – will help ensure an acceptable quality of life for all, protect wildlife and be ecologically sustainable.

The projected population rise would, if historic trends were followed, be accompanied by a significant rise in global consumption of meat and dairy products, with some predictions indicating a potential doubling in consumption of these products by 2050. The problem, however, is that increasing the number of animals reared and slaughtered globally, from the present approximately seventy billion farmed land animals, has several important consequences on a planet with finite resources.

First, all of these animals must eat. Ideally, ruminants such as sheep and cattle would graze land that could not be used to grow crops for people. This would allow nutritional benefit to be derived from such land, and the livestock would be complementary to food crops elsewhere. Under some circumstances, the grazed land could even extract and store atmospheric carbon, in a process known as carbon sequestration. But with so many animals, including non-grazing animals such as the world's billions of pigs and poultry, land of this kind is insufficient. Instead, crops must be grown specifically for feeding to these animals, so rainforests and other biodiverse regions such as the Brazilian Cerrado (a vast area of tropical savannah) are being cleared, both to create grazing land for cattle and to grow crops such as soy for animal feed. Around 30 per cent of former rainforest areas cleared for animal agriculture have been converted to cropland, especially soy, growing feed for the world's cattle, pigs, poultry and fish.

Because of these devastating changes of land use (and the loss of plants and animals that accompany it), together with other environmental impacts, such as transporting feed across the world and the reliance of feed crops on fossil-fuel-based fertilizer, the global livestock system accounts for an estimated 14.5 per cent of human-caused greenhouse gas emissions. The figure masks regional variations and does not separate out the impacts of different greenhouse gases, but it is accepted that global animal agriculture can be a significant contributor to environmental degradation, climate change and biodiversity loss.

From an animal welfare perspective, meeting such high demand for animal-derived food while mitigating these environmental consequences may tend towards a demoralizing assumption that further intensification would be required to minimize carbon footprints – more confinement, more barren environments, higher yields and faster growth rates, with the consequences outlined in previous chapters. Ironically, at the moment in history when science has finally given insights into the nature of animal wellbeing and suffering, guiding us towards a need for greater compassion, issues facing the future of humanity would seem, at first glance, to have transpired against this. Or have they?

If the recommendations provided by organizations such as Population Matters become more widely considered, the human population rise itself may not turn out to be so dramatic. But even if the rise is as great as currently predicted, the accompanying nutrition transition towards a higher meat and dairy intake not only poses risks to the planet's ability to support human life, but it also has negative health implications. While some animal-derived foods in our diet can be beneficial, a higher level of consumption of red meat and processed red meat (such as bacon, hot dogs and sausage) in Western diets is associated with increased risk of cardiovascular disease and certain types of cancer. Medical bodies including Public Health England and the UK's National Health Service recommend an average maximum daily intake of red and processed meat of 70 grams per day. Globally, almost double the optimal amount of processed meat is consumed. In the UK, around a third of the population is reported to eat more than the recommended healthy amount of meat. Taking these impacts together, the UK Health Alliance on Climate Change – which includes medical, nursing and veterinary royal colleges, faculties of health, the British Medical Association, the *British Medical Journal* and *The Lancet* – is urging health professionals to help their patients to improve their health and lower their greenhouse gas emissions by encouraging them to eat less meat.

These health concerns are set against the backdrop of a world in which nearly 690 million people are hungry, while over 650 million are obese. There is not a lack of food in the world, but an inequitable distribution of nutrients across the face of the planet.

Ninety-nine per cent of our history as humans was spent as hunter-gatherers, hunting wild animals and gathering wild plants, until the advent of farming. During this long ancestral period, we evolved to enjoy eating nutritionally valuable sugar and fat, increasing our desire to eat them when they were available. Now, like domesticated animals, this motivation is another remnant of an evolutionary past which struggles to find meaningful expression in the modern world. Previously, our food supply was seasonal; now, in the developed world, we have constant access to almost any food we want. Sugary and fatty foods sell well, as we struggle to resist them when they are made available. As Professor Jimmy Bell, obesity specialist at Imperial College, London, is quoted as saying, 'Genetically, human beings haven't changed, but our environment, our access to cheap food has.'

It is within our collective scientific ken that consuming these foods in excess contributes to obesity and lowered life expectancy, and that the agricultural methods which produce our food are jeopardizing the planet's ability to accommodate us. And yet, as individuals and as a society, we struggle to act. Despite our intelligence and capacity for wisdom, the production and consumption of food remind us of our frailty.

As was highlighted in Chapter 3, farmers produce products that people will buy. This may sound obvious, but it is important to remember. The vast majority of farmers care and are concerned about how animals are treated. But as has been demonstrated, many of our farming systems, though operated with compassion, are intrinsically incapable of achieving a good life for animals. Let us assume that a given farmer accepts that, say, the painfully lame broilers or the crated pigs are suffering and the situation is unacceptable. A farmer whom I once met expressed the sentiment of many: 'I'm as keen to see this improved as you, but do you know how much it would cost to change? I'd give each of my animals golden slippers if someone would pay for the product.'

In its 2011 Report on Economics and Farm Animal Welfare, FAWC stated that it 'deplores the low profitability of livestock farming'. In the 1960s, UK households typically spent 20 per cent of their income on food and drink. Now, around 10 per cent is typical. Following the Second World War, agricultural policy was directed at producing more and cheaper food, so prices have gone down and consumption has risen.

It is clear that if we select products on price alone we will seek the lowest prices, in order to afford other things. I am influenced in this way like everybody else. But animal-derived foods have become cheaper at the expense of the animals' welfare.

One important problem is that many people do not know what type of production system their meat, eggs or dairy products have come from. If they knew an animal had had a life that they would not condone, they might pay a little extra, rather than shop on price alone. Among European citizens, 59 per cent say they are willing to pay more for products from 'animal welfare-friendly production systems' and 57 per cent of US citizens said they would be likely to choose a restaurant because it serves welfare-certified animal products. And some will realize that this is not just a matter of avoiding such products on principle. They realize that in buying lower-welfare products, they fund those who are treating animals that way; they are actually rewarding the low-welfare practices with their own money.

Currently, there is still too little information made available to citizens on which they can base their decisions. Economist Professor Richard Bennett and his colleagues found that 72 per cent of UK respondents were concerned about the welfare of farmed animals, but only 38 per cent felt well informed about how they are treated. Europe-wide, 64 per cent of citizens said they would like to have more information about the conditions under which farmed animals are treated in their country. This book has aimed to give some of that information, including how we know what is important for animals. But wider education and discussion is needed on all areas of animal use, the benefits of a healthy natural environment, the imperative to tackle antimicrobial resistance, which is driven through irresponsible prescribing of antibiotics in people and animals, and the undeniable connections between these topics and the overall wellbeing of ourselves and our planet. The global One Health and One Welfare approaches – which foster interdisciplinary collaboration between veterinary, human health and environmental professionals and others – are underpinned by recognition that the health and wellbeing of people, animals and the environment are linked. As one example, approximately 75 per cent of emerging infectious diseases around the world are zoonoses (diseases that can be transmitted from animals to humans) and most of them are driven by human activities and our impacts on the environment. Future pandemic prevention and preparedness has a critical dependence on rapidly expanded One Health working.

If citizens are aware of issues arising from differing farming practices (or even if we are simply aware that our purchases can be kinder to animals), we can then look for logos on food packets that assure higher standards. Several schemes now exist internationally, including the RSPCA Assured scheme, Soil Association organic, the British Red Tractor scheme, Global Animal Partnership in the US, the French Label Rouge scheme, Beter leven in the Netherlands and the Bioland label in Germany.

Of the UK schemes, the Red Tractor logo assures that animals have been reared in accordance with British legal requirements, or beyond the legal minimum in some cases, allowing consumers to avoid the worst animal welfare practices that are not legally permissible in Britain. It ensures stunning prior to slaughter and a slightly reduced stocking density for meat chickens, for example, but permits farrowing crates for sows and cages for laying hens.

The RSPCA Assured scheme goes further, beyond basic industry standards, through its own higher welfare standards, designed to address the most important welfare problems affecting each species of farmed animal. For example, it does not permit farrowing crates and cages for laying hens.

Organic food offers assurances against a number of sustainability goals including building soil fertility rather than depending on artificial fertilizers, high levels of on-farm biodiversity and high standards of animal welfare. Organically farmed animals are slower growing or lower yielding, housed at lower stocking densities and able to express important elements of their normal behaviour through a more natural lifestyle. Like RSPCA Assured, close confinement systems such as crates and cages are not permitted.

Recently, both the European Commission and the UK government have, separately, announced their intentions to reform animal welfare labelling 'to make it easier for consumers to purchase food that aligns with their welfare values'. To help now, the British Veterinary Association has produced a downloadable #ChooseAssured infographic (see the appendix, page 292) to help shoppers recognize and understand the main UK food assurance schemes.

With reliable information and trustworthy logos, we can reward farmers who are going further to make more humane farming a reality. Shopping in this way for meat, eggs and dairy products is one of the simplest ways for individuals to effect change. UK sales of ethical food and drink, including organic and RSPCA Assured, have increased year on year since 2007, despite the economic downturn, and now account for around 11 per cent of all household food sales.

Because of the power of ethical consumption, logos have also been developed to allow us to act on other ethical concerns, in addition to animal welfare. For example, the Marine Stewardship Council (MSC certified) logo aims to assure that fish have been harvested from sustainable stocks; the Rainforest Alliance logo, applied to products such as tea and coffee, offers assurances around conservation of biodiversity and sustainable livelihoods for people; while the Fairtrade scheme assures improved access to markets for disadvantaged farmers and workers in developing countries. A number of years ago I was inconsistent in my approach to seeking higher-welfare logos when shopping for food (and, undoubtedly, sometimes still am). I doubted that such an action would make any meaningful difference to the problems I was concerned about, unconvinced that sufficient numbers of others would do the same. But I came to realize that with this uncertainty was a worse certainty – that if I bought lower-welfare products, I was directly funding and rewarding those who were producing them. My money was validating the simple assertion that 'we are only producing what the public wants': the words that disturbed Ruth Harrison as she wrote *Animal Machines* in 1964, and echo to this day.

Many people assume that higher-welfare products are more costly than they actually are. As we saw in Chapter 4, some budget supermarkets are now leading stockists of RSPCA Assured products. The UK government's Department for the Environment, Food & Rural Affairs reports that the average UK household with children spends £60 per month on food that could have been eaten but was thrown away. UK householders are already spending money that could be used to support higher standards of animal welfare, but it is going straight into the bin.

In 2012, the cost to save all of the world's globally threatened species – including mammals, amphibians, reptiles and birds – was estimated at around £3 billion a year: less than half of Europe's annual expenditure on ice cream. Martin Harper, former Conservation Director of the Royal Society for the Protection of Birds (RSPB), reported in 2018 that we spend five times more a year on pet care products (US $103 billion) worldwide than we do on the entire global network of protected nature areas (US $22 billion).

The disparity in welfare standards tolerated for farmed animals versus companion animals is also expressed in economic terms. US sales of pet treats are today reported to be worth an estimated US $6 billion, having increased by 29 per cent in the five years to 2017. UK dog treats continued a decade-long growth trend to £462 million, attributed to, among other factors, the increasing humanization of pets. In the UK 91 per cent of dog owners give their pets treats and 81 per cent of cat owners do the same, but Chapter 11 drew attention to the pet obesity epidemic, now affecting over 60 per cent of pet dogs in the UK. For millions of UK pet owners, stopping or reducing feeding commercial pet treats, and allocating the saved money to higher animal welfare meat and dairy products for the family, would achieve a double animal welfare benefit – reducing the risk of pet obesity while directly funding improvements to the lives of farmed animals. The science of human behaviour change is increasingly being applied to social challenges such as this, including in animal welfare – recognizing that simply sharing knowledge or factual insights is often insufficient and that understanding how and why people make the decisions they do is critical.

Similarly, the less-and-better approach to consumption of meat and dairy, promoted by the British Veterinary Association among others, recommends reducing consumption of animal-derived foods while maintaining the amount that is spent on them. They suggest paying a little more for a smaller overall quantity, so that these foods are properly valued and farmers rewarded for their ethical husbandry and environmental stewardship. In the UK, flexitarianism – where people choose to eat meat less frequently – has become increasingly popular, and there has been growing media coverage of plant-based food initiatives such as Veganuary (in which people try veganism for the month of January). Twenty-one per cent of British people are looking to cut down on their red meat consumption and investors are said to view the market in meat and dairy alternatives (such as meat-free burgers) as a key prospect.

Ways of achieving social change, such as improved environmental and animal welfare standards, include our purchasing decisions, retailers' corporate social responsibility policies (aiming to 'do the right thing'), retailers' brand protection policies (aiming to not be found 'doing the wrong things'), education of young people and government policies such as taxation, public spending and legislation.

Supermarkets, like any business, seek to provide their customers with what they want. If a shop provides everything that we, as shoppers, want, then we will have every reason to visit that shop. If a retailer perceives its customers to want improved animal welfare standards, then they will respond by stocking higher-welfare products. But how do they know what their customers want? Whenever I have asked retailers this question, the answer has been that they primarily respond to demand. That is, if higher-welfare products fly off their shelves, this signals an appetite for such products and the retailer will stock more. But notice that the responsibility here has returned to us, the shoppers. If enough of us purchase this way, then retailers might take the decision to edit their range, by stopping selling certain lower-welfare products. But they are unlikely to do that without first having gauged customer support for alternatives.

A circumstance in which retailers might take such a decision without first gauging customer demand is in the case of pressure from animal welfare charities. Here, again, we might breathe a sigh of relief that a third party is acting on our concerns. But many charities are entirely reliant on charitable funding and must pursue campaigns that achieve their charitable objectives as well as attract supporters. If we, as citizens, do not engage with the charities' work – for example, by signing petitions, becoming a member or making a donation – then we have failed to signal to that charity that we would like their work in a particular area to continue.

Retailers may sometimes elect to support higher animal welfare standards as part of their commitment to corporate social responsibility, but if they do not perceive this to be important to their customer base, animal welfare may be afforded low priority relative to other environmental and social concerns. The Business Benchmark on Farm Animal Welfare, produced annually since 2012, was the first report to objectively and independently examine farm animal welfare policies within the food industry, to provide information for investors and others on key animal welfare issues and risks. It has recognized the leadership being demonstrated by food businesses such as Marks & Spencer and Waitrose, and now covers 150 companies across 25 countries. Many companies are still providing limited information on their farm animal welfare performance, but in the 2020 Benchmark, 23 companies had moved up at least one tier and the overall average score continued to increase, to 35 per cent in 2020 from 25 per cent in 2012.

Where retailers are taking proactive steps, this can be highlighted and championed by animal welfare charities. For example, the Compassion in World Farming Good Farm Animal Welfare Awards recognize food companies that are implementing positive farm animal welfare policies across their supply chains, such as researching and trialling alternatives to farrowing crates. Conversely, charities can shine a spotlight on bad practice and if this resonates with consumers, businesses can change their practices rapidly (and often in ways that they had previously argued were impossible). Following lobbying on gestation crates (sow stalls) by the Humane Society of the United States (HSUS), a number of high-profile US food businesses, including McDonald's, Wendy's and Kraft Foods have committed to eliminating gestation crate confinement of pigs through their supply chains.

As well as signalling our desires through higher-welfare purchases, we can also ask at restaurants and other food retail outlets whether higher-welfare options are available, or could be made available in future. Business managers often interpret such requests as being representative of a wider proportion of their customers.

Finally, there are many who feel that if a production system cannot prevent animal suffering, or enable an animal to experience a good life, it should not be legal. Responsibility for animal welfare, they feel, should be the job of government. Governments can establish minimum standards of animal welfare, below which a majority of the population would judge welfare to be unacceptable or to be described as cruel. In this way, minimum legal standards represent a lowest common denominator and may not be as aspirational as some private initiatives. But they can prevent the worst practices, especially when applied internationally, such as the EU-wide bans on veal crates in 2006, barren battery cages in 2012 and sow stalls in 2013. Businesses may also look to government to create national and international legislation, so that they are not outcompeted when there are costs associated with improving standards. As well as legislation, as we saw in Chapter 5 with the introduction of England's Animal Health and Welfare Pathway, government funding can be allocated to provide much-needed investment for progressive and ambitious animal health and welfare goals.

But governments, like businesses and NGOs, need to know that their policies will be supported. Politicians in a democracy need to win votes and are driven to promote policies that will appeal to the electorate. Again, we are back to the actions of the informed and concerned citizen – each and every one of us. Just as we must signal our desires to retailers through our purchases (or abstention) or customer feedback, we should also contact our local elected representatives on matters that concern us, or look for animal welfare and environmental policies during election campaigns so that we can reward them with our vote.

At whichever level positive change can occur, it is down to us as individuals to make our desires known and to persuade others to do the same. This individual action is not *instead* of action by corporations, retailers, governments and others; rather it is part of stimulating and supporting the necessary transformative action across society.

My purpose, following on from the work begun by Ruth Harrison in 1964 and reinforced by others since, has simply been to sketch a reminder of what happens to those animals who are currently used for human benefit across the world, together with the underpinning evidence of animal welfare impacts. It is important to reiterate that this science can only tell us what is, not what should be. Science does not answer our ethical questions, but provides us with relevant facts. Ultimately, value judgements are called upon from each of us to ensure that society affords a standard of care for animals that we are collectively comfortable with and can be proud of. I cannot dictate what these judgements should be, but recognizing that responsibility falls to each of us, the following gives examples of practical actions we could take.

Personal

- Look for logos when food shopping that support higher-welfare farming (e.g. RSPCA Assured), sustainable harvest of fish (e.g. MSC certified) and environmental protection and sustainable livelihoods (e.g. Rainforest Alliance). Use guides such as the British Veterinary Association's #ChooseAssured infographic (see page 292) to help you.

- If you eat these foods, eat less and better meat and dairy; for example, limiting meat to two to three times a week (unless medical advice says otherwise), and using the saved money to buy meat, eggs and dairy products with higher animal welfare and environmental attributes.

- If dining out, choose a restaurant that offers higher-welfare options.

- If you are fortunate to have a garden, keep wildlife in mind when gardening. UK gardens cover an area larger than all of the country's national nature reserves combined, so the potential for benefiting wildlife is substantial. Wildlife-rich gardens, with flowers for bees, butterflies and other pollinators, can be beautiful and calming. Various wildlife charities provide free guides on wildlife-friendly gardening.

- If you are concerned about the welfare of animals used in sport, do not bet on, or attend, these sporting events.

- If you are thinking of getting a pet, ask for advice about which type to get at your local veterinary practice. Then, for puppies or kittens, download the free puppy contract and puppy information pack or kitten checklist. They will help you ask the right questions to ensure the young animal is healthy and has been raised with kindness.

- Take the time to train your pet, ideally by attending well-run training classes, to build your relationship with them and help them understand how you want them to behave. It is never too late to start, but basic reward-based training can start at around six weeks of age. Never use dominance-based methods. Animal training instructors who use kind, effective methods can be found on the website of the Animal Behaviour and Training Council. The charity Dogs Trust offers its low-cost Dog School training classes, which use reward-based methods, across the UK.

- If your pet develops a problem behaviour, contact an animal behaviourist registered through the Animal Behaviour and Training Council – this ensures that practitioners are using humane, evidence-based techniques. First, seek veterinary advice to rule out a possible medical cause, such as pain.

- The Energy Saving Trust provides free information on improving efficiencies around the home.

- You can offset your carbon emissions (for example, following an unavoidable flight) by donating to a reputable carbon-offsetting scheme.

- Donate to, become a member of and/or support the campaigns of a charity that is working to address your concerns. The charities mentioned in this book are all doing valuable work and are dependent on public support.

- Talk about your concerns with others and influence them through your positive actions. Social scientists point out that behaviour change should be made as fun and hopeful as possible; people and organizations who are too pessimistic are often dismissed as doomsters.

To influence businesses

- Ask at restaurants about the welfare standards of the animals who have provided their meat, either during your visit or in a customer satisfaction survey afterwards.

- If your workplace provides staff catering, enquire about sustainability assurances such as animal welfare and the sourcing of local products (note that these are separate – local does not necessarily mean higher welfare). You could encourage them, perhaps by collaborating with similarly minded colleagues, to join the Food for Life Served Here scheme, which helps restaurants and caterers demonstrate their commitment to healthy and ethical food.

- Instigate or support workplace energy and environmental initiatives, such as recycling, switching lights off or cycling to work. In the veterinary profession, a recently launched Greener Veterinary Practice Checklist is supporting veterinary practices to become more sustainable – perhaps your area of work has something similar?

To influence governments

- Write to your local elected representative, either to raise a concern or to feed your comments into an existing topic of discussion. If you live in the UK, you can easily find your local MP, with contact details, at www.theyworkforyou.com

- Participate in campaigns, for example, by signing online petitions or sharing messages and videos via social media. When I attended meetings on the EU wild bird trade, the European Commissioner commented that he had received thousands of campaigning postcards at his office, supporting a permanent import ban. This activity had been coordinated by the campaigning organization Eurogroup for Animals and proved to me that such activities – which would now be social media campaigns – are noticed.

It was time to turn back and I lowered myself down from the fence. The woodland was just as quiet, just as remote. I took a deep breath and felt its refreshing earthy perfume rush into my lungs. My senses reactivated and I started treading slowly back along the path. The surrounding peace was still only disturbed by the faint, high-pitched calls of distant tits or occasional finches flying overhead. A trilling party of long-tailed tits appeared in the canopy and rippled through its branches.

I rounded the final bend in the path, back towards my car. I had enjoyed my dawn visit, marrying a morning's thoughts to the optimism of the rising sun. Then, ahead, I once again saw movement, this time at the end of a stretch of wire fence. My heart was beating, as there had been something different about what I had just seen. I scanned the binoculars slowly from the wire across to each surrounding leaf and back. Then I saw a spindly twig bouncing as though it had just been danced upon. I flicked the binoculars back to the wire. As I did, a minute bird appeared, their tiny claws gripped around the woven wire. The bird was animated, vanishing into the shrubbery, then back again. But they were moving towards me and I could make out a perfect white line painted above the eye. The bird's back was olive-green, with bright greenish-yellow on the side of their neck and a bronze blush finishing off their pale flanks. In a single shaft of sunlight, now beaming through the trees like a spotlight on a high-wire, the tiny bird's golden crown shone through my clutched lenses.

This was a firecrest: a tiny ball of hand-painted feathers, weighing a vanishing six grams, skipping along the wire, jumping across tufts of lichen and plucking tiny spiders from their webs. With the bird fixed by the glare of the sun and my watching eyes, I was now locked into fleeting seconds of pleasure which subverted my entire sense of time and place, temporarily sealing off the entire contents of my mind. Now, all of my capacity to be enthralled and affected by the natural world – my geese-filled sunsets, bejewelled hummingbirds, blowing whales, seabirds spilling from soaring cliffs, chorusing toads, tumbling lapwings, perfect orchids, sweeping falcons and the golden sand dunes where my heart will forever reside –

was blazing within this dainty creature. The fire-capped kinglet. They teetered to within ten metres of my frozen position, hovered to glean one final insect from a soft clump of moss and then permanently disappeared into the sprawling undergrowth as quickly as they had appeared.

The natural world inspires and informs. For me, the world of animals is a world of beauty and suffering. The distinction is, of course, entirely false because life in the natural world is, as Thomas Hobbes said, 'nasty, brutish and short'. But the mind generalizes; wild nature becomes a source of beauty, breeding moral concern for its preservation, while humanity's impositions on other animals become sources of suffering, generating grave concerns for their welfare. Acting on both concerns will be essential for our own continued wellbeing and that of our world. Motivating factors will include economics, but I, like many, am moved by the aesthetic and inspirational appeal of wild animals and landscapes. The migrations that connect us with global communities; the intricate and complex behaviour and plumage that spark our wonder and fascination; the wild music of haunting and beautiful calls and songs; the astonishing creation of nests – such as the firecrest's, which can take three weeks to construct and will hang from the tip of a branch – a tiny, deep cup of moss and spider's web, lined with feathers, including a final carefully arranged few that will provide an overarching insulating parasol. And there is the constancy of natural rhythms in our lives, connecting us to a universe in which life on earth is predicted to end through the heat of our ageing sun in a billion years, but in which preventable animal and human suffering is a daily reality.

Nature's beauty offers space in which to think and reflect but also acts as a buffer, offsetting some of the terrible pity generated by our treatment of other animals. For each depth to which occurrences of institutionalized animal suffering have plunged me, a subsequent wild spectacle has served to elevate and recalibrate my dampened spirit. Nothing is predetermined, and how animals and our natural environment are treated is in our hands. We are small in the face of the world's many and complex problems, but with the firecrest came a powerful reminder of the impact of every tiny individual.

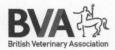

#ChooseAssured
UK Farm Assurance
Schemes Infographic

	Farm Assured Welsh Livestock	Lion Eggs Code of Practice
Please note that this list of the BVA's welfare priorities is not exhaustive and these priorities will be addressed and assessed differently across the different schemes. The level of welfare achieved across the different schemes may vary. For more detailed information about the different standards and requirements used by farm assurance schemes please visit their respective websites.		
Animals are stunned before slaughter	Assurance does not cover slaughter	Assurance does not cover slaughter
Veterinary involvement Veterinary professionals are involved in livestock health planning and review	✓	✓
Prohibit environments that substantially reduce behavioural opportunity Enriched cages for laying hens Farrowing crates for sows (pre-birth until weaning)	N/A – Scheme only applies to beef and lamb	Permits enriched cages for laying hens
Support responsible use of antimicrobials	✓	✓
Animal health and biosecurity Measures to protect animal health and prevent the spread of disease	✓	✓
Lifetime assurance Animals spend their whole lives on an assured farm, livestock transport is assured ie. standards assure the management of health and welfare during transportation and scheme has standards to ensure welfare at slaughter**	Assurance does not cover slaughter	Assurance does not cover slaughter
Measures to protect the environment ie. guidance on preventing environmental contamination, pollution and minimising waste	✓	✓

**Schemes may address some of these areas even if products are not lifetime assured.

Below is a reference grid that sets out BVA priorities for farm animal* welfare against what is addressed in the standards of different UK farm assurance schemes. Products may be assured by more than one of these schemes or an assurance scheme not addressed in this graphic. Please check the label of food products carefully.

As part of the #ChooseAssured campaign, BVA is encouraging the veterinary profession and the wider public to #ChooseAssured by purchasing UK animal-derived products that are farm assured. Through the campaign we're raising awareness of the great work of the UK's farm assurance schemes and the crucial work of vets within the schemes to safeguard high animal health and welfare.

*including farmed fish

Northern Ireland Beef and Lamb Farm Quality Assurance Scheme	Quality Meat Scotland	Red Tractor	RSPCA Assured	Soil Association
Assurance does not cover slaughter	✓	✓	✓	✓
✓	✓	✓	✓	✓
N/A – Scheme only applies to beef and lamb	Permits farrowing crates for sows (pre-birth until weaning)	Permits farrowing crates for sows (pre-birth until weaning)	✓	✓
✓	✓	✓	✓	✓
✓	✓	✓	✓	✓
Assurance does not cover slaughter	✓	Pigs and meat poultry only	All species except dairy – dairy calves can be sourced from non-assured farms	Assurance does not cover transport
✓	✓	✓	Farmed salmon and trout only	✓

Last reviewed: January 2019, Review date: 2022

* More information about BVA's #ChooseAssured campaign, together with a full-colour, downloadable version of the #ChooseAssured infographic, is available at https://www.bva.co.uk/take-action/choose-assured-farm-assurance-campaign/

Notes

Chapter 1 — Beneath the skin

One of the first, and most famous, scientists — Darwin C. *On the Origin of Species by Means of Natural Selection, or the Preservation of Favoured Races in the Struggle for Life.* John Murray, 1859

the colourful textbook — Young B, Woodford P and O'Dowd G. Preface to the First Edition of *Wheater's Functional Histology*, 6th edition, *A Text and Colour Atlas.* Churchill Livingstone, 2013

pain, fear, comfort and enjoyment — Scottish Animal Welfare Commission: statement on animal sentience, 2021. www.gov.scot/publications/scottish-animal-welfare-commission-statement-on-animal-sentience/ (Accessed 8th August 2021)

six thousand or so mammalian species — Burgin CJ, Colella JP, Kahn PL et al. How many species of mammals are there? *Journal of Mammalogy* 99 (2018), 1–14. https://doi.org/10.1093/jmammal/gyx147

visit the online mammalian brain museum — Comparative mammalian brain collections. The University of Wisconsin, Michigan State University and the National Museum of Health and Medicine. www.neurosciencelibrary.org (Accessed 8 August 2021)

Brain-imaging studies of guinea pigs — Panksepp J. Feeling the pain of social loss. *Science* 302 (2003), 237–9.

if a ewe is viewing her lamb — See: Kendrick K. Quality of life and the evolution of the brain. *Animal Welfare* 16 (2007), 9–15

suffer dread about what might happen — Kirkwood JK, Hubrecht R. Animal Consciousness, Cognition and Welfare. *Animal Welfare* 10 (2001), 5–17

some aspects of the suffering of clever animals might be less — Broom D. Quality of life means welfare: How is it related to other concepts and assessed? *Animal Welfare* 16 (2007), 45–53

University of Lincoln cold-blooded cognition lab — www.lincoln.ac.uk/home/ lifesciences/research/animalbehaviourcognitionandwelfare/animalcognition/ (Accessed 8 August 2021)

In Hugh's Chicken Run *'— Hugh's Chicken Run'* — KEO Films, 3 episodes, presented by Hugh Fearnley-Whittingstall, 2008

display signs of empathy ¢ Edgar JL, Lowe JC, Paul ES et al. Avian maternal response to chick distress. *Proceedings of the Royal Society B: Biological Sciences* 278 (2011), 3129–34

Cambridge Declaration on Consciousness — The Cambridge Declaration on Consciousness was publicly proclaimed in Cambridge, UK, on 7 July 2012 at the Francis Crick Memorial Conference on Consciousness in Human and non-Human Animals, at Churchill College, University of Cambridge

Crustacean Compassion — Do crabs and lobsters feel pain? Scientific evidence presented by Crustacean Compassion: www.crustaceancompassion.org.uk/do-crustaceans-feel-pain (Accessed 8 August 2021)

An independent review published in November 2021 — Birch J, Burn C, Schnell A et al. *Review of the Evidence of Sentience in Cephalopod Molluscs and Decapod Crustaceans*. London School of Economics and Political Science, 2021

Verlyn Klinkenborg wrote — Klinkenborg, V. Darwin at 200: the ongoing force of his unconventional idea. *Opinion, New York Times*, 11 February 2009: www. nytimes.com/2009/02/12/opinion/12thu4.html (Accessed 8 August 2021)

Pythagoras — Ovid, *The Teachings of Pythagoras*. Republished as pages 367–79 in *Ovid's Metamorphoses* (R Humphries, translator). Indiana University Press, 1955. Cited in Fraser D. *Understanding Animal Welfare – The Science in its Cultural Context*. Wiley-Blackwell, 2008

William Blake ('A Robin Red breast...') — Blake W, *Auguries of Innocence*, 1863

The eminent animal welfare lawyer — Radford M. Informed debate: the contribution of animal welfare science to the development of public policy. *Animal Welfare* 13:4 (2004), 171–4

Animal Machines — Harrison R. *Animal Machines*. Vincent Stuart, 1964

appointed a committee — Brambell FWR (chairman). *Report of the Technical Committee to Enquire into the Welfare of Animals kept under Intensive Livestock Husbandry Systems*. Her Majesty's Stationery Office, 1965

conglomerate concept' — Discussed in Fraser D. *Understanding Animal Welfare: The Science in its Cultural Context*, Chapter 11 — How do the different measures relate to each other? Wiley-Blackwell, 2008

The resulting Five Freedoms — Cited in *Farm Animal Welfare in Great Britain: Past, Present and Future.* Farm Animal Welfare Council, 2009

The Five Domains — Mellor DJ, Beausoleil NJ, Littlewood KE et al. The 2020 Five Domains model: Including human–animal Interactions in assessments of animal welfare. *Animals* 10 (2020), 1870. https://doi.org/10.3390/ani10101870

The Animal Welfare Acts of 2006 and the Welfare of Animals Act 2011 in Northern Ireland — Animal Welfare Act 2006; Animal Health and Welfare (Scotland) Act 2006; Welfare of Animals Act (Northern Ireland) 2011

Each of us has an animal welfare footprint — Veterinarian Dr James Yeates introduced the concept of an animal welfare footprint in Yeates J. *Animal Welfare in Veterinary Practice.* Wiley-Blackwell, 2013

over a billion are reared for food — *Agriculture in the United Kingdom 2020.* Department for Environment, Food and Rural Affairs. www.gov.uk/government/statistics/agriculture-in-the-united-kingdom-2020 (Accessed 10 August 2021)

over 70 billion globally — *FAOSTAT.* Food and Agriculture Organization of the United Nations

Interest in vegetarianism and veganism — E.g. *Consumer Insights: The Rise of Plant-Based Food Products and Implications for Meat and Dairy.* Agriculture and Horticulture Development Board, 2018

— See also Interest in veganism is surging. *The Economist* 29 January 2020. www.economist.com/graphic-detail/2020/01/29/interest-in-veganism-is-surging (Accessed 1 October 2021)

meat produced from cell culture — E.g. Would you eat meat grown from cells in a laboratory? Here's how it works. *The Conversation* 23 June 2019. https://theconversation.com/would-you-eat-meat-grown-from-cells-in-a-laboratory-heres-how-it-works-117420 (Accessed 10 August 2021)

one of the six highest-ranking countries — Animal Protection Index. https://api.worldanimalprotection.org/#

Chapter 2 — Australian zebra finches

estimated at £210 million a year — Pet Food Manufacturers' Association Data Report 2018. https://www.pfma.org.uk/_assets/docs/annual-reports/PFMA-Pet-Data-Report-2018.pdf (Accessed 14 August 2021)

contributory source of endangerment — Wild Bird Trade and CITES. https://www.birdlife.org/worldwide/policy/wild-bird-trade-and-cites (Accessed 14 August 2021)

'highly social and mobile lives' — Zann RA. *The Zebra Finch: A Synthesis of Field and Laboratory Studies.* Oxford University Press, 1996

24 per cent of their waking time — Wensley SP, Nevison CM and Stockley P. The behaviour and welfare of zebra finches under typical pet shop conditions.

Proceedings of the 35th International Congress of the ISAE. Center for Animal Welfare at UC Davis, 2001

added to the UK red list — Eaton MA, Aebischer NJ, Brown et al. Birds of Conservation Concern 4: The population status of birds in the United Kingdom, Channel Islands and Isle of Man. *British Birds* 108 (2015), 708–46

Although there are behavioural differences — Jensen P (ed.). *The Ethology of Domestic Animals: An Introductory Text.* CABI Publishing, 2017

Domestic animals are not man-made — Dawkins MS. Behavioural deprivation: A central problem in animal welfare. *Applied Animal Behaviour Science* 20: 3–4 (1988), 209–25. https://doi.org/10.1016/0168-1591(88)90047-0

The pigs, despite being domesticated — Fraser D. *Understanding Animal Welfare: The Science in its Cultural Context.* Wiley-Blackwell, 2008

When keeping animals in captivity — Berdoy M. *The Laboratory Rat: A Natural History.* 2002. https://www.youtube.com/watch?v=giu5WjUt2GA (Accessed 14 August 2021)

In the early 1980s, Dawkins developed — (1) Dawkins MS. Battery hens name their price: Consumer demand theory and the measurement of ethological 'needs', *Animal Behaviour* 31:4 (1983), 1195–205. doi.org/10.1016/S0003-3472(83)80026-8

— (2) Dawkins MS. Behavioural deprivation: A central problem in animal welfare, *Applied Animal Behaviour Science* 20:3–4 (1988), 209–25. doi.org/10.1016/0168-1591(88)90047-0

— (3) From an animal's point of view: Motivation, fitness and animal welfare. *Behavioral and Brain Sciences* 13 (1990), 1–61

An experiment with American mink — Mason GJ, Cooper J and Clarebrough C. Frustrations of fur-farmed mink. *Nature* 410 (2001), 35–6. doi:10.1038/35065157

if given a pre-formed nest — Arey DS, Petchey AM and Fowler VR. The preparturient behaviour of sows in enriched pens and the effect of pre-formed nests. *Applied Animal Behaviour Science* 31:1–2 (1991), 61–68

When male guinea pigs are separated — Sachser N, Dürschlag M and Hirzel D. Social relationships and the management of stress. *Psychoneuroendocrinology* 23:8 (1998), 891–904. doi:10.1016/s0306-4530(98)00059-6

researchers studying canaries — Sargent TD and Keiper RR. Stereotypies in caged canaries. *Animal Behaviour* 15 (1967), 62–6. doi.org/10.1016/S0003-3472(67)80012-5

researchers studying zebra finches — Jacobs H, Smith N, Smith P et al. Zebra finch behaviour and effect of modest enrichment of standard cages. *Animal Welfare* 4 (1995), 3–9 *it is surprising that* — Nager RG and Law G. The zebra finch. In Hubrecht R and Kirkwood J (eds). *The UFAW Handbook on the Care and Management of Laboratory and Other Research Animals,* 8th edition. Wiley-Blackwell, 2010

The charm of these birds — *The Wild Places of Essex*. AGB Films for BBC NHU/Discovery Channel/BBC Worldwide. Written and narrated by Robert MacFarlane, 2010

Chapter 3 — Herons and hens

a quarter of UK adults — Research by Linking Environment And Farming (LEAF), in 'Do you know where bacon comes from', *Daily Express,* 1 June 2017. https://www.express.co.uk/news/uk/675831/British-produce-meat-bacon-beef-milk-eggs-farms-UK (Accessed 14 August 2021)

a quarter of 8–11 year old children — British Nutrition Foundation, reported by Farming UK, 12 June 2017. https://www.farminguk.com/news/british-children-lack-basic-food-knowledge-survey-shows_46677 (Accessed 14 August 2021)

Approximately half of the laying hens in Europe — Kollenda E, Baldock D, Hiller N and Lorant A. *Transitioning towards Cage-free Farming in the EU: Assessment of Environmental and Socio-economic Impacts of Increased Animal Welfare Standards*. Policy report by the Institute for European Environmental Policy, Brussels and London, 2020

equating to over 175 million birds — Eggs. European Commission ('There are more than 350 million laying hens in the European Union'). https://ec.europa.eu/info/food-farming-fisheries/animals-and-animal-products/animal-products/eggs_en (Accessed 14 August 2021)

36 per cent of eggs — Department for the Environment, Food and Rural Affairs. Quarterly UK statistics about eggs — statistics notice (data to June 2021). https://www.gov.uk/government/statistics/egg-statistics/quarterly-uk-statistics-about-eggs-statistics-notice-data-to-june-2021 (Accessed 14 August 2021)

the UK's 39 million laying hens — Countrysideonline.co.uk. About the industry. https://www.countrysideonline.co.uk/food-and-farming/feeding-the-nation/eggs/#:~:text=There%20are%2039%20million%20commercial%20laying%20hens%20in%20the%20UK (Accessed 14 August 2021). See also *Agriculture in the UK 2020*, p. 20. Department for Environment, Food and Rural Affairs.

to house around 4.5 billion — *Egg Track 2020 Report*. Compassion in World Farming, 2020

approximately 7.5 billion laying hens globally — Food and Agriculture Organization of the United Nations, FAOSTAT. Cited in *Egg Track 2020 Report*. Compassion in World Farming, 2020

70 per cent of laying hens in the US (over 200 million birds in cages) — United States Department of Agriculture Egg Markets Overview, March 2020

— The Humane Society of the United States states: 'The vast majority of egg-laying hens in the United States are confined in battery cages'. https://www.humanesociety.org/resources/cage-free-vs-battery-cage-eggs (Accessed 14 August 2021)

66 per cent of laying hens in Canada (17 million birds in battery cages) — (1) Egg farming in Canada. The British Columbia Society for the Prevention of Cruelty to Animals. https://spca.bc.ca/programs-services/farm-animal-programs/farm-animal-production/egg-laying-hens/ (Accessed 14 August 2021)

— (2) 26 million laying hens in Canada. Egg fact sheet. Farm and Food Care, Ontario, 2016. https://www.farmfoodcareon.org/wp-content/uploads/2017/05/Hen-and-Egg-fact-sheet-2016final.pdf (Accessed 14 August 2021)

half of laying hens in Australia — National flock size of 20,946,659 layers in June 2019. Australian Eggs. https://www.australianeggs.org.au/egg-industry (Accessed 14 August 2021)

11 million birds in battery cages. The Poultry Site, 28 November 2019. https://www.thepoultrysite.com/news/2019/11/research-reveals-aussie-shoppers-unaware-of-caged-egg-industry (Accessed 14 August 2021)

over 90 per cent of laying hens in China — Hartcher K. *Supporting High Welfare Cage-free Egg Production in China. Guidance Memo prepared for the Tiny Beam Fund.* 2020

world's biggest egg producer — Global egg production continues to rise. *Poultry World,* 29 June 2020. https://www.poultryworld.net/Eggs/Articles/2020/6/Global-egg-production-continues-to-rise-604164E/ (Accessed 14 August 2021)

2.8 billion birds in cages — Table 1: Number of laying hens in China, 2018. Wu Y and Qin F. Analysis on production efficiency of laying hens in China—based on the survey data of five provinces. *Journal of Agricultural Science* 11 (2019), 280. doi.org/10.5539/jas.v11n8p280

Approximately 30 million chicks are killed — Policy position on surplus male production animals. British Veterinary Association, British Cattle Veterinary Association, Goat Veterinary Society and British Veterinary Poultry Association, 2019. https://www.bva.co.uk/media/3098/bva-bcva-bvpa-gvs-surplus-male-animals-position-oct-2019.pdf (Accessed 14 August 2021)

Before the females are ten days old — Policy position on feather pecking in laying hens. British Veterinary Association and British Veterinary Poultry Association, 2019. https://www.bva.co.uk/media/3696/bva-and-bvpa-policy-position-on-feather-pecking-in-laying-hens.pdf (Accessed 14 August 2021)

estimated to afflict approximately half of all laying hens — An open letter to Great Britain Governments: keel bone fractures in laying hens. Farm Animal Welfare Committee, 16 August 2013. https://assets.publishing.service.gov.uk/

government/uploads/system/uploads/attachment_data/file/324505/FAWC_advice_on_keel_bone_fractures_in_laying_hens.pdf (Accessed 14 August 2021)

one of the most important welfare problems — *Opinion on Osteoporosis and Bone Fractures in Laying Hens.* Farm Animal Welfare Council, December 2010. https://assets.publishing.service.gov.uk/government/uploads/system/uploads/attachment_data/file/325043/FAWC_opinion_on_osteoporosis_and_bone_fractures_in_laying_hens.pdf (Accessed 14 August 2021)

whether housed in cages or not — Position paper on moving towards more animal welfare friendly systems for laying hens. Federation of Veterinarians of Europe, 11 June 2021. https://fve.org/cms/wp-content/uploads/002-Welfare_friendly_systems_Laying-Hens-draft_adopted.pdf (Accessed 14 August 2021)

This is a collective term used to describe — What is feather pecking? FeatherWel. https://www.featherwel.org/featherwel/injuriouspecking.html (Accessed 14 August 2021)

associated with stress and boredom — Policy position on feather pecking in laying hens. British Veterinary Association and British Veterinary Poultry Association, 2019. https://www.bva.co.uk/media/3696/bva-and-bvpa-policy-position-on-feather-pecking-in-laying-hens.pdf (Accessed 14 August 2021)

risk factors include — IBID

Professors Jonathan Cooper and Michael Appleby — Cooper JJ and Appleby MC. Demand for nest boxes in laying hens. *Behavioural Processes* 36:2 (1996), 171–82. doi 10.1016/0376-6357(95)00027-5

Dr Anna Olsson and Professor Linda Keeling — Olsson IA and Keeling LJ. Night-time roosting in laying hens and the effect of thwarting access to perches. *Applied Animal Behaviour Science* 68:3 (2000), 243–56. doi: 10.1016/s0168-1591(00)00097-6.

Olsson and Keeling conducted a second series of experiments — Olsson IA, Keeling LJ. The push-door for measuring motivation in hens: Laying hens are motivated to perch at night. *Animal Welfare* 11 (2002), 11–19

a large EU-funded project on the welfare of laying hens — Advantages and disadvantages of different housing systems for the welfare of laying hens. LayWel – Welfare implications of changes in production systems for laying hens. https://www.laywel.eu/web/xmlappservlet7bc1.html?action (Accessed 14 August 2021)

With increased knowledge — Rogers LJ. *The Development of Brain and Behaviour in the Chicken.* CAB International, 1995, p. 213

It has long been believed — Weeks CA, Lambton SL and Williams AG. Implications for welfare, productivity and sustainability of the variation in reported levels of mortality for laying hen flocks kept in different housing systems: A meta-analysis of ten studies. *PloS ONE* 11:1 (2016), e0146394. https://doi.org/10.1371/journal.pone.0146394

a large-scale study — Schuck-Paim C, Negro-Calduch E and Alonso WJ. Laying hen mortality in different indoor housing systems: a meta-analysis of data from commercial farms in 16 countries. *Scientific Reports* 11 (2021), 3052. https://doi.org/10.1038/s41598-021-81868-3

'Good Life potential' — (1) — Adapted from the concept of 'welfare potential'. Lymbery P. The theory and application of welfare potential. In *Proceedings of the Importance of Farm Animal Welfare Science to Sustainable Agriculture Forum*. Beijing: CIWF, RSPCA, WSPA, HSI with the support of the European Commission, 2008

— (2) Further information on Good Life and laying hen welfare. Edgar JL, Mullan SM, Pritchard JC et al. Towards a 'Good Life' for farm animals: Development of a resource tier framework to achieve positive welfare for laying hens *Animals* 3 (2013), 584–605. https://doi.org/10.3390/ani3030584

The view of the Federation of Veterinarians of Europe — Position paper on moving towards more animal welfare friendly systems for laying hens. Federation of Veterinarians of Europe, 11 June 2021. https://fve.org/cms/wp-content/uploads/002-Welfare_friendly_systems_Laying-Hens-draft_adopted.pdf (Accessed 14 August 2021)

together with the European Food Safety Authority — EFSA Panel on Animal Health and Welfare (AHAW). Scientific Opinion on the Welfare of Laying Hens on Farm. *EFSA Journal*. 2023; EFSA Journal 2023; 21(2): 7789.

doi: 10.2903/j.efsa.2023.7789

In 1998, just 21 per cent of eggs — *The Welfare State: Measuring Animal Welfare in the UK 2008*, RSPCA, 2009, p. 42

today it is 58 per cent — Department for the Environment, Food and Rural Affairs. Quarterly UK statistics about eggs — statistics notice (data to June 2021) https://www.gov.uk/government/statistics/egg-statistics/quarterly-uk-statistics-about-eggs-statistics-notice-data-to-june-2021 (Accessed 14 August 2021)

identify and destroy male embryos prior to hatching — (1) Policy position on surplus male production animals. British Veterinary Association, British Cattle Veterinary Association, Goat Veterinary Society and British Veterinary Poultry Association. 2019. https://www.bva.co.uk/media/3098/bva-bcva-bvpa-gvs-surplus-male-animals-position-oct-2019.pdf (Accessed 14 August 2021)

identify and destroy male embryos prior to hatching — (2) FVE position on killing unwanted offspring in farm animal production. Federation of Veterinarians of Europe, 15 November 2017. https://www.fve.org/cms/wp-content/uploads/045-Surplus-animals_adopted.pdf (Accessed 14 August 2021)

Chapter 4 — Sea cliffs and chickens

around 1 billion chickens are slaughtered — *Agriculture in the United Kingdom 2020.* Department for Environment, Food and Rural Affairs. www.gov.uk/government/ statistics/agriculture-in-the-united-kingdom-2020 (Accessed 15 August 2021)

approximately 66 billion — *FAOSTAT.* Food and Agriculture Organization of the United Nations

In the 1950s — EFSA Panel on Animal Health and Welfare (AHAW). Scientific opinion on the influence of genetic parameters on the welfare and the resistance to stress of commercial broilers. *EFSA Journal* 8:7 (2010), 1666. doi:10.2903/j. efsa.2010.1666

up to 100 grams of weight every single day — Butterworth, A. Cheap as chicken. In D'Silva J and Webster J (eds). *The Meat Crisis,* 2nd edition. Earthscan, 2017

painful lameness, affecting millions — Granquist E, Vasdal G, De Jong I et al. Lameness and its relationship with health and production measures in broiler chickens. *Animal* 13:10 (2019), 2365–72. doi:10.1017/S1751731119000466

In a study that assessed the walking ability — Knowles TG, Kestin SC, Haslam S et al. Leg disorders in broiler chickens: Prevalence, risk factors and prevention. *PloS ONE* 3 (2008), e1545. doi:10.1371/journal.pone.0001545

Figures from Norway — Granquist E, Vasdal G, De Jong I et al. Lameness and its relationship with health and production measures in broiler chickens. *Animal* 13:10 (2019), 2365–72. doi:10.1017/S1751731119000466

study published in the Veterinary Record — McGeown D, Danbury TC, Waterman-Pearson A et al. Effect of carprofen on lameness in broiler chickens. *Veterinary Record* 144 (1999), 668–71. 10.1136/vr.144.24.668

In a second study — Danbury TC, Weeks C, Chambers JP et al. Self-selection of the analgesic drug carprofen by lame broilers. *Veterinary Record* 146 (2000) 307–11. 10.1136/vr.146.11.307

jostle with one another more frequently — Stamp Dawkins M, Donnelly C and Jones T. Chicken welfare is influenced more by housing conditions than by stocking density. *Nature* 427 (2004), 342–4. doi.org/10.1038/nature02226

disturbed when attempting to rest — Hall A. The effect of stocking density on the welfare and behaviour of broiler chickens reared commercially. *Animal Welfare* 10 (2001), 23–40

European Union's Scientific Committee on Animal Health and Animal Welfare (SCAHAW) concluded — *The Welfare of Chickens Kept for Meat Production (Broilers).* Scientific Committee on Animal Health and Animal Welfare (SCAHAW). European Commission, Health and Consumer Protection Directorate-General, 2000

a European Union Directive — Council Directive 2007/43/EC of 28 June 2007 laying down minimum rules for the protection of chickens kept for meat production

UK government codes of practice — e.g. *Code of Practice for the Welfare of Meat Chickens and Meat Breeding Chickens*. Department for Environment, Food and Rural Affairs, 2018

Following a substantial review — Scientific Opinion on the welfare of broilers on farm. EFSA Journal. 2023; 21(2): 7788. doi: 10.2903/j.efsa.2023.7788

highlighted by the European Food Safety Authority (EFSA)'s Panel on Animal Health and Welfare — EFSA Panel on Animal Health and Welfare (AHAW). Scientific opinion on the influence of genetic parameters on the welfare and the resistance to stress of commercial broilers *EFSA Journal* 8:7 (2010), 1666. doi:10.2903/j.efsa.2010.1666

described by EFSA as a 'widespread problem' — IBID. For review of prevalence data, see also Hartcher KM and Lum HK. Genetic selection of broilers and welfare consequences: a review. *World's Poultry Science Journal* 76 (2020), 154–67, doi: 10.1080/00439339.2019.1680025

typically comprising 2,500–3,000 birds — EFSA Panel on Animal Health and Welfare (AHAW). Scientific opinion on welfare aspects of the management and housing of the grand-parent and parent stocks raised and kept for breeding purposes. *EFSA Journal* 8:7 (2010), 1667. doi:10.2903/j.efsa.2010.1667

abnormally functioning ovaries and poor fertility — Hocking PM (ed.), Feed restriction. In *Biology of breeding poultry*. CABI, 2009

peck in their empty feeders and at the non-nutritive litter — Merlet F, Puterflam J, Faure JM et al. Detection and comparison of time patterns of behaviours of two broiler breeder genotypes fed ad libitum and two levels of feed restriction. *Applied Animal Behaviour Science* 94 (2005), 255–71

described as 'rough' — EFSA Panel on Animal Health and Welfare (AHAW). Scientific Opinion on welfare aspects of the management and housing of the grand-parent and parent stocks raised and kept for breeding purposes. *EFSA Journal* 8:7 (2010), 1667. doi:10.2903/j.efsa.2010.1667

EFSA suggest that genetic selection — de Jong I, Berg C, Butterworth A et al. Scientific report updating the EFSA opinions on the welfare of broilers and broiler breeders. *Supporting Publications*, 2012, EN-295

studies suggest that mechanical catching — Duncan IJH, Slee GS, Kettlewell P et al. Comparison of the stressfulness of harvesting broiler chickens by machine and by hand. *British Poultry Science* 27:1 (1986), 109–114, doi: 10.1080/00071668608416861

Specifically, they recommend a maximum — Scientific Opinion on the welfare of broilers on farm. *EFSA Journal*. 2023; 21(2): 7788.

doi: 10.2903/j.efsa.2023.7788

even if this objective may require – EFSA Panel on Animal Health and Welfare (AHAW). Scientific opinion on the influence of genetic parameters on the welfare and the resistance to stress of commercial broilers. *EFSA Journal* 8:7 (2010), 1666, *doi:10.2903/j. efsa.2010.1666*

even if this may involve [reducing...] – EFSA Panel on Animal Health and Welfare (AHAW). Scientific opinion on welfare aspects of the management and housing of the grandparent and parent stocks raised and kept for breeding purposes. *EFSA Journal* 8:7 (2010), 1667, doi:10.2903/j.efsa.2010.1667

Soil Association organic standards — 3.12.2 Number of birds permitted in each house. *Soil Association Farming and Growing Standards 2021.* Soil Association, 2021

increased by 54 per cent — More than half of shoppers recognise RSPCA Assured label. 2019. https://business.rspcaassured.org.uk/press-and-media/more-than-half-of-shoppers-recognise-rspca-assured-label/ (Accessed 15 August 2021)

the Better Chicken Commitment — https://betterchicken.org.uk/ (Accessed 15 August 2021)

An independent commercial-scale trial — Rayner AC, Newberry RC, Vas J et al. Slow-growing broilers are healthier and express more behavioural indicators of positive welfare. *Scientific Reports* 10 (2020), 15151. doi.org/10.1038/s41598-020-72198-x

a 2021 study — Luuk SM, Vissers HW, Saatkamp AGJM, et al. Analysis of synergies and trade-offs between animal welfare, ammonia emission, particulate matter emission and antibiotic use in Dutch broiler production systems. *Agricultural Systems* 189 (2021), doi.org/10.1016/j.agsy.2021.103070

a KFC spokesperson said — The European Chicken Commitment and KFC – FarmGate podcast with Jenny Packwood, Director of Responsibility and Reputation for KFC UK and Ireland, and Annie Rayner and Kelly Watson, experts in broiler systems and behaviour, working at FAI Farms. https://www.faifarms.com/podcasts/european-chicken-commitment-and-kfc/ (Accessed 15 August 2021)

Chapter 5 — Orchids and pigs

16 million turkeys — Number of turkeys slaughtered annually in the United Kingdom (UK) from 2003 to 2020. https://www.statista.com/statistics/298320/turkey-slaughterings-in-the-united-kingdom-uk-by-breed/ (Accessed 18 August 2021)

around 10 million of whom — Pate E. Farm turkeys still a winner at Christmas — with over 10 million sold in UK. *Farmers Guardian*, 22 December 2019. https://www.fginsight.com/news/news/farm-turkeys-still-a-winner-at-christmas---with-over-10-million-sold-in-uk-99923 (Accessed 18 August 2021)

estimated EU average litter size — 2019 *Pig Cost of Production in Selected Countries*. Agriculture and Horticulture Development Board, 2021

They have well-developed social and cognitive abilities — (1) Mendl M, Held S and Byrne R. Pig cognition. *Current Biology* 20 (2010), R796–8. doi:10.1016/j. cub.2010.07.018

— (2) Nawroth C, Langbein J, Coulon M et al. Farm animal cognition – linking behavior, welfare and ethics. *Frontiers in Veterinary Science* 6 (2019), 24. 10.3389/ fvets.2019.00024

Nest building is a highly motivated behaviour — Arey DS, Petchey AM and Fowler VR. The preparturient behaviour of sows in enriched pens and the effect of pre-formed nests. *Applied Animal Behaviour Science* 31 (1991), 61–8

among nearly quarter of a million — Derived from: (1) *UK Pig Facts and Figures, 2019*. Agriculture and Horticulture Development Board, 2019

(2) Government urged not to rush into banning farrowing crates, 11 March 2021. https://www.pig-world.co.uk/news/government-urged-not-to-rush-into-banning-farrowing-crates.html (Accessed 18 August 2021)

(3) *Proposals for Public Goods Payments for Farm Animal Welfare*. Farm Animal Welfare Forum, 2020

a third of all meat consumed — Global pork market forecast (2018 to 2026) – by production, consumption, import, export & company. https://www. globenewswire.com/news-release/2020/05/12/2031727/0/en/Global-Pork-Market-Forecast-2018-to-2026-By-Production-Consumption-Import-Export-Company.html (Accessed 18 August 2021)

around 143 million farmed in the European Union — Eurostat 2020. Cited in: Kollenda E, Baldock D, Hiller N et al. *Transitioning Towards Cage-free Farming in the EU: Assessment of Environmental and Socio-economic Impacts of Increased Animal Welfare Standards*. Policy report by the Institute for European Environmental Policy, Brussels and London, 2020

approximately 10 million are slaughtered each year — *UK Pig Facts and Figures, 2019*. Agriculture and Horticulture Development Board, 2019

approximately 409,000 — IBID

around 12 per cent of piglets born indoors — IBID

The Federation of Veterinarians of Europe's view — Position paper on moving towards more welfare-friendly farrowing systems. Federation of Veterinarians of Europe and European Association of Porcine Health Management, 12 November 2021. https://fve.org/cms/wp-content/uploads/FVE-position-paper-on-moving-towards-more-welfare-friendly-farrowing-systems_adopted. pdf (Accessed 4 December 2021)

The International Veterinary Students' Association — Position statement on the European Citizens' Initiative 'End the Cage Age'. International Veterinary

Students' Association. 2021. https://ivsaanimalwelfarecommittee.wordpress.com/2021/03/23/position-statement-of-the-international-veterinary-students-association-on-the-european-citizens-initiative-end-the-cage-age/ (Accessed 18 August 2021)

often lacks suitable material to forage and root in — (1) Nalon E and De Briyne N. Efforts to ban the routine tail docking of pigs and to give pigs enrichment materials via EU law: Where do we stand a quarter of a century on? *Animals* 9 (2019), 132. doi.org/10.3390/ani9040132

— (2) *Real Welfare Update Report, 2018–2020.* Agriculture and Horticulture Development Board, 2021

more likely to display 'teeth champing' — Noonan GJ, Rand JS, Priest J et al. Behavioural observations of piglets undergoing tail docking, teeth clipping and ear notching. *Applied Animal Behaviour Science* 39:3–4(1994), 203–13

histopathological evidence — Hay MJ, Rue C, Sansac G et al. Long term detrimental effects of tooth clipping or grinding in piglets: An histological approach. *Animal Welfare* 13 (2004), 27–32

after tail docking, these behaviours — Noonan GJ, Rand JS, Priest J et al. Behavioural observations of piglets undergoing tail docking, teeth clipping and ear notching. *Applied Animal Behaviour Science* 39:3–4 (1994), 203–13

Only around 2 per cent of piglets — Highlighting the differences – how UK welfare standards compare with our competitors. 5 May 2017. https://www.pig-world.co.uk/news/highlighting-the-differences-how-uk-welfare-standards-compare-with-our-competitors.html (Accessed 18 August 2021)

In a Canadian study — Taylor AA and Weary DM, Vocal response of piglets to castration: identifying procedural sources of pain. *Applied Animal Behaviour Science* 70 (2000), 17–26

A separate study — White RG, DeShazer JA, Tressler CJ et al. Vocalization and physiological response of pigs during castration with or without a local anesthetic. *Journal of Animal Science* 73 (1995), 381–6

docked tail stumps often contain — *Opinion on Pig Mutilations and Environmental Enrichment in Piglets and Growing Pigs.* Farm Animal Welfare Council, 2011

a 'high proportion' of indoor-kept piglets — IBID

72 per cent of pigs — *Real Welfare Update Report, 2018–2020.* Agriculture and Horticulture Development Board. 2021

estimated 7 million pigs per year — *Proposals for Public Goods Payments for Farm Animal Welfare.* Farm Animal Welfare Forum, 2020

The British Veterinary Association supports — BVA position on UK sustainable animal agriculture. British Veterinary Association, 2019. https://www.bva.co.uk/media/1181/bva-position-on-uk-sustainable-animal-agriculture-full.pdf (Accessed 18 August 2021)

including most of the US, Canada and Brazil — Pig welfare standards – unpicking the differences. 14 October 2019. https://www.adas.uk/News/pig-welfare-standards-unpicking-the-differences (Accessed 19 August 2021)

urinary tract infections linked to their chronic inactivity — *The Welfare of Intensively Kept Pigs.* Report of the Scientific Veterinary Committee of the European Commission, 1997

less frequently in the first few days — IBID

the European Union passed a Directive — Council Directive 2008/120/EC (the Pigs Directive) of 18 December 2008 laying down minimum standards for the protection of pigs

but the legislation is often ignored — Nalon E and De Briyne N. Efforts to ban the routine tail docking of pigs and to give pigs enrichment materials via EU law: Where do we stand a quarter of a century on? *Animals* 9 (2019), 132

but most countries illegally continue to do so — De Briyne N, Berg C, Blaha T et al. Phasing out pig tail docking in the EU — present state, challenges and possibilities. *Porcine Health Management* 4 (2018), 27. doi.org/10.1186/s40813-018-0103-8

Finland, Norway, Sweden and Switzerland — Position on preventing tail docking and tail biting. Federation of Veterinarians of Europe and European Association of Porcine Health Management, 2019

repetitive infringements — Nalon E and De Briyne N. Efforts to ban the routine tail docking of pigs and to give pigs enrichment materials via EU law: Where do we stand a quarter of a century on? *Animals* 9 (2019), 132

the proportion is generally lower — *Opinion on Pig Mutilations and Environmental Enrichment in Piglets and Growing Pigs.* Farm Animal Welfare Council, 2011

King Solomon's Ring — Lorenz, K. *King Solomon's Ring.* 1949

around 40 per cent of breeding sows — Highlighting the differences – how UK welfare standards compare with our competitors. 5 May 2017. https://www.pig-world.co.uk/news/highlighting-the-differences-how-uk-welfare-standards-compare-with-our-competitors.html (Accessed 19 August 2021)

most of the remaining 60 per cent — UK Government response to petition: *End the Cage Age for all farmed animals.* 20 August 2021. https://petition.parliament.uk/petitions/593775?reveal_response=yes (Accessed 7 October 2021)

See also RSPCA Assured – pigs. https://www.rspcaassured.org.uk/farm-animal-welfare/pigs/ (Accessed 19 August 2021)

around 96 per cent — Pig welfare standards – unpicking the differences. 14 October 2019. https://www.adas.uk/News/pig-welfare-standards-unpicking-the-differences (Accessed 19 August 2021)

pig product labels — IBID

agroforestry approaches — See e.g. *Farming for Change – Mapping a Route to 2030.* Food, Farming and Countryside Commission, 2021

a comprehensive review published in 2021 — Åkerfeldt MP, Gunnarsson S, Bernes G et al. Health and welfare in organic livestock production systems – a systematic mapping of current knowledge. *Organic Agriculture* 11 (2021), 105–32. doi. org/10.1007/s13165-020-00334-y

go little beyond minimum legal standards — Pig welfare standards – unpicking the differences. 14 October 2019. https://www.adas.uk/News/pig-welfare-standards-unpicking-the-differences (Accessed 19 August 2021)

Chapter 6 — Goose days

half a million pink-footed geese — Brides K, Mitchell C and Auhage SNV. *Status and Distribution of Icelandic-breeding Geese: results of the 2019 International Census.* Wildfowl & Wetlands Trust, 2020

South-west Lancashire is visited — IBID

International Consensus Principles for Ethical Wildlife Control — Dubois S, Fenwick N, Ryan EA et al. International consensus principles for ethical wildlife control. *Conservation Biology* 31:4 (2017), 753–60. doi: 10.1111/cobi.12896

elephants in Africa and Asia — Shaffer LJ, Khadka KK, Van Den Hoek J et al. Human–elephant conflict: A review of current management strategies and future directions. *Frontiers in Ecology and Evolution* 6 (2019), 235. Doi: 10.3389/fevo.2018.00235

'culture of coexistence' — Dubois S, Fenwick N, Ryan EA et al. International consensus principles for ethical wildlife control. *Conservation Biology* 31:4 (2017), 753–60. doi: 10.1111/cobi.12896

'compassionate conservation' — e.g. Beausoleil NJ. I am a compassionate conservation welfare scientist: Considering the theoretical and practical differences between compassionate conservation and conservation welfare. *Animals* 10:2 (2020), 257. doi.org/10.3390/ani10020257

instant and prolonged distress — Mason GJ and Littin KE. The humaneness of rodent pest control. *Animal Welfare* 12 (2003), 1–37

mouths becoming glued shut — Fenwick N. *Evaluation of the Humaneness of Rodent Capture Using Glue Traps – prepared for the Canadian Association of Humane Trapping.* CAHT, 2013

more humane alternative methods — Guiding principles in the humane control of rats and mice. Universities Federation of Animal Welfare (UFAW). www.ufaw.org.uk/rodent-welfare/rodent-welfare (Accessed 19 August 2021)

including...the British Veterinary Association — Policy position on the use and sale of rodent glue traps. British Veterinary Association and British Veterinary Zoological Society, 2021. https://www.bva.co.uk/media/4362/full-bva-position-on-the-use-and-sale-of-rodent-glue-traps.pdf (Accessed 4 December 2021) *the UK government announced* — *Our Action Plan for Animal Welfare.* Department for Environment, Food and Rural Affairs, 2021

In 2022, the UK government banned — Glue Traps (Offences) Act 2022

Chapter 7 — Robins and cows

an estimated 95,000 male dairy calves — Policy position on surplus male production animals. British Veterinary Association, British Cattle Veterinary Association, Goat Veterinary Society and British Veterinary Poultry Association, 2019. https://www.bva.co.uk/media/3098/bva-bcva-bvpa-gvs-surplus-male-animals-position-oct-2019.pdf (Accessed 20 August 2021)

Until 2007 in the European Union — Council Directive 97/2/EC of 20 January 1997 amending Directive 91/629/EEC laying down minimum standards for the protection of calves

promoting the benefits of higher welfare [British] rose veal — Policy position on surplus male production animals. British Veterinary Association, British Cattle Veterinary Association, Goat Veterinary Society and British Veterinary Poultry Association, 2019. https://www.bva.co.uk/media/3098/bva-bcva-bvpa-gvs-surplus-male-animals-position-oct-2019.pdf (Accessed 20 August 2021)

See also Policy position on killing unwanted offspring in farm animal production. Federation of Veterinarians of Europe, 2017. https://www.fve.org/cms/wp-content/uploads/045-Surplus-animals_adopted.pdf (Accessed 20 August 2021)

sales of sexed semen doubling — *Sexed Semen Sales Double.* Agriculture and Horticulture Development Board, 2021

industry-led GB Dairy Calf Strategy — GB Dairy Calf Strategy 2020–2023. National Farmers' Union and Agriculture and Horticulture Development Board

return to normal within two hours — Petrie NJ, Mellor DJ, Stafford KJ et al. Cortisol responses of calves to two methods of disbudding used with or without local anaesthetic. *New Zealand Veterinary Journal* 44:1 (1996), 9–14. doi: 10.1080/00480169.1996.35924

heart rate stays higher than in control calves — IBID

A calf's behaviour supports this conclusion — Stafford K and Mellor DJ. Dehorning and disbudding distress and its alleviation in calves. *Veterinary Journal* 169 (2005), 337–49. doi:10.1016/j.tvjl.2004.02.005

Further research indicates — Ede T, Lecorps B, von Keyserlingk MAG et al. Calf aversion to hot-iron disbudding. *Scientific Reports* 9 (2019), 5344. doi.org/10.1038/s41598-019-41798-7

not have to be a vet to perform disbudding — e.g. *Code of Recommendations for the Welfare of Livestock: Cattle.* Department for Environment, Food and Rural Affairs

perception of, and willingness to treat, pain — Remnant JG, Tremlett A, Huxley JN et al. Clinician attitudes to pain and use of analgesia in cattle: where are we 10 years on? *Veterinary Record* 181 (2017), 400. doi.org/10.1136/vr.104428

The British Veterinary Association (BVA), together with — Policy statement on analgesia in calves. British Veterinary Association and British Cattle Veterinary Association, 2017 https://www.bva.co.uk/media/1172/analgesia-in-calves.pdf (Accessed 20 August 2021)

as does the American Association of Bovine Practitioners — *Dehorning Guidelines.* American Association of Bovine Practitioners, 2019 https://aabp.org/Resources/ AABP_Guidelines/Dehorning-2019.pdf (Accessed 20 August 2021)

BVA and BCVA are calling for — Policy statement on analgesia in calves. British Veterinary Association and British Cattle Veterinary Association, 2017 https:// www.bva.co.uk/media/1172/analgesia-in-calves.pdf (Accessed 20 August 2021)

described as one of the most pressing issues — (1) Griffiths BE, Grove White D and Oikonomou G. A cross-sectional study into the prevalence of dairy cattle lameness and associated herd-level Risk factors in England and Wales. *Frontiers in Veterinary Science* 5 (2018), 65. doi: 10.3389/fvets.2018.00065

— (2) *Position on Welfare of Dairy Cows: Lameness.* Federation of Veterinarians of Europe, 2019 https://fve.org/cms/wp-content/uploads/002-FVE-position-cattle-lameness_adopted.pdf (Accessed 20 August 2021)

affects approximately a third — IBID

equivalent to around three-quarters of a million — Red Tractor review missed opportunity for change. The VetPartners Mobility Special Interest Group. *Vet Times*, 2 March 2021

now produces over 8,000 litres — *UK Milk Yield.* Agriculture and Horticulture Development Board, 2021. https://ahdb.org.uk/dairy/uk-milk-yield (Accessed 20 August 2021)

The European Food Safety Authority's — Scientific Opinion of the Panel on Animal Health and Welfare on a request from European Commission on the overall effects of farming systems on dairy cow welfare and disease. *EFSA Journal* 1143 (2009), 1–38

lost more than half of its dairy farmers — Uberoi E. *UK Dairy Industry Statistics.* Briefing Paper, House of Commons Library, 2020

several veterinary commentators — e.g. Huxley J and Green M. More for less: dairy production in the 21st century. *Veterinary Record* 167:18 (2010), 712–3. doi: 10.1136/vr.c5676

New purpose-built units — IBID

In an advisory letter — FAWC letter to UK Minister, Jim Paice: The welfare of dairy cows housed all year round and/or in very large herds. 4 August 2010

strong motivation to access pasture — von Keyserlingk M, Amorim Cestari A, Franks B et al. Dairy cows value access to pasture as highly as fresh feed. *Scientific Reports* 7 (2017), 44953. doi.org/10.1038/srep44953

indicators of improved emotional wellbeing — Crump A, Jenkins K, Bethell EJ et al. Optimism and pasture access in dairy cows. *Scientific Reports* 11 (2021), 4882. doi. org/10.1038/s41598-021-84371-x

We hope that our research — Cows with no pasture may have 'damaged emotional wellbeing'. *Farming UK*, 18 March 2021. https://www.farminguk.com/news/ cows-with-no-pasture-may-have-damaged-emotional-wellbeing-_57822.html (Accessed 20 August 2021)

Federation of Veterinarians of Europe advocating — *Position on Welfare of Dairy Cows: Lameness.* Federation of Veterinarians of Europe, 2019. https://fve.org/ cms/wp-content/uploads/002-FVE-position-cattle-lameness_adopted.pdf (Accessed 20 August 2021)

Ninety-five per cent of the British public — Studies for UK, Germany, United States, Canada and Brazil, cited in Crump A, Jenkins K, Bethell EJ et al. Optimism and pasture access in dairy cows. *Scientific Reports* 11 (2021), 4882. doi.org/10.1038/ s41598-021-84371-x

worldwide, most milk now — Scientific opinion on welfare of dairy cows in relation to behaviour, fear and pain based on a risk assessment with special reference to the impact of housing, feeding, management and genetic selection. European Food Safety Authority. *EFSA Journal* 7 (2009), 1139

less than 5 per cent of the 10 million — von Keyserlingk M, Amorim Cestari A, Franks B et al. Dairy cows value access to pasture as highly as fresh feed. *Scientific Reports* 7 (2017), 44953. doi.org/10.1038/srep44953

Sweden, where full-time housing — Van den Pol-van Dasselaar A, Hennessy D, Isselstein J. Grazing of dairy cows in Europe – an in-depth analysis based on the perception of grassland experts. *Sustainability* 12:3 (2020), 1098

around 95 per cent of UK dairy cows — *Opinion on the Welfare of Cattle Kept in Different Production Systems.* Animal Welfare Committee, 2021

a growing proportion of dual-purpose dairy cattle are being bred — Policy position on surplus male production animals. British Veterinary Association, British Cattle Veterinary Association, Goat Veterinary Society and British Veterinary Poultry Association, 2019. https://www.bva.co.uk/media/3098/bva-bcva-bvpa-gvs-surplus-male-animals-position-oct-2019.pdf (Accessed 20 August 2021)

Another approach is to mate dairy cows — Rutherford NH, Lively FO and Arnott G. A review of beef production systems for the sustainable use of surplus male dairy-origin calves within the UK. *Frontiers in Veterinary Science* 8 (2021), 388. doi: 10.3389/fvets.2021.635497

Global Animal Partnership 5-step — The Global Animal Partnership 5-step Animal Welfare Rating Program. www.globalanimalpartnership.org/5-step-animal-welfare-rating-program (Accessed 20 August 2021)

Business Benchmark — Amos N, Sullivan R and Williams R. *The Business Benchmark on Farm Animal Welfare Report.* BBFA, 2020, www.bbfaw.com/media/1942/bbfaw-report-2020.pdf (Accessed 20 August 2021)

Chapter 8 — Starlings and slaughter

travel around 30 miles — Summers RW and Feare CJ. Roost departure by European starlings *Sturnus vulgaris*: Effects of competition and choice of feeding site. *Journal of Avian Biology* 26:4 (1995) 289–95

They are amongst the most popular — Bateson M and Asher L. The European Starling. In Hubrecht R and Kirkwood J (eds). *The UFAW Handbook on the Care and Management of Laboratory and Other Research Animals*; 8th edition. Wiley-Blackwell, 2010

The experimental starlings were first trained — Matheson S, Asher L and Bateson M. Larger, enriched cages are associated with 'optimistic' response biases in captive European starlings (*Sturnus vulgaris*). *Applied Animal Behaviour Science* 109 (2008), 374–83. 10.1016/j.applanim.2007.03.007

investigated abnormal repetitive behaviour — Brilot BO, Asher L and Bateson M. Stereotyping starlings are more 'pessimistic'. *Animal Cognition* 13:5 (2010), 721–31. doi: 10.1007/s10071-010-0323-z

'avoidable pain, distress or suffering' — UK and EU legislation laid out in: Position on the welfare of animals at slaughter. British Veterinary Association, 2020. https://www.bva.co.uk/media/3664/full-position-bva-position-on-the-welfare-of-animals-at-slaughter.pdf (Accessed 21 August 2021)

Farm Animal Welfare Committee (now Animal Welfare Committee) concluded — (1) *Report on the Welfare of Animals at Slaughter or Killing Part 1: Red Meat Animals.* Department for Environment, Food and Rural Affairs, 2003

— (2) *Report on the Welfare of Farmed Animals at Slaughter or Killing Part 2: White Meat Animals.* Department for Environment, Food and Rural Affairs, 2009

research using electroencephalography — Examples of such research:

(1) Gibson TJ, Johnson CB, Murrell JC et al. Electroencephalographic responses of halothane-anaesthetised calves to slaughter by ventral neck incision without prior stunning. *New Zealand Veterinary Journal* 57:2 (2009), 77–83

(2) Gibson TJ, Johnson CB, Murrell JC et al. Amelioration of electroencephalographic responses to slaughter by non-penetrative captive bolt stunning after ventral neck incision in halothane anaesthetised calves. *New Zealand Veterinary Journal* 57:2 (2009), 96–101

The Federation of Veterinarians of Europe — Position on slaughter of animals without prior stunning. Federation of Veterinarians of Europe, 2002. https://fve.org/cms/wp-content/uploads/fve_02_104_slaughter_prior_stunning.pdf (Accessed 21 August 2021)

Chapter 9 — Skylarks and sheep

To many humans — Kendrick K. Sheep senses, social cognition and capacity for consciousness. In Dwyer C (ed.). *The Welfare of Sheep*. Springer, 2008

In 2001, these findings were published — Kendrick K, Costa A, Leigh A et al. Sheep don't forget a face. *Nature* 414 (2001), 165–6. 10.1038/35102669

interested in the brain regions — Kendrick KM and Baldwin BA. Cells in temporal cortex of conscious sheep can respond preferentially to the sight of faces. *Science* 24 April 1987, pp. 448–50

recognise different emotions — Tate AJ, Fischer H, Leigh AE et al. Behavioural and neurophysiological evidence for face identity and face emotion processing in animals. *Philosophical Transactions of the Royal Society of London* 361:1476 (2006), 2155–72. doi:10.1098/rstb.2006.1937

shown in profile — Kendrick KM, Leigh A, Peirce J. Behavioural and neural correlates of mental imagery in sheep using face recognition paradigms. *Animal Welfare* 10:S1 (2001), 89–101

approximately 30 million sheep — Total number of sheep and lambs in June 2020 was 32.7 million. https://ahdb.org.uk/news/uk-sheep-flock-numbers-revised-downward (Accessed 22 August 2021)

approximately 3 million sheep lame — Opinion on Lameness in Sheep. Farm Animal Welfare Council. Department for Environment, Food and Rural Affairs, 2011

willingness or ability to catch and treat — Kaler J and Green L. Recognition of lameness and decisions to catch for inspection among sheep farmers and specialists in GB. *BMC Veterinary Research* 4 (2008), 41. doi.org/10.1186/1746-6148-4-41

It also disadvantages the farmer — IBID

the 'five-point plan' — Clements R, Stoye S. The 'Five Point Plan': A successful tool for reducing lameness in sheep. *Veterinary Record* (2014), 175. 10.1136/vr.102161

national prevalence in the UK flock — Best CM, Roden J, Pyatt AZ et al. Uptake of the lameness Five-Point Plan and its association with farmer-reported lameness prevalence: A cross-sectional study of 532 UK sheep farmers. *Preventive Veterinary Medicine* 181 (2020), 105064. doi.org/10.1016/j.prevetmed.2020.105064

72 per cent of farmers would now treat — IBID

there is an optimism — Reilly B. Reducing lameness in the national flock – a never-ending story? *Veterinary Practice*. 1 March 2021. https://www.veterinary-practice.com/article/reducing-lameness-in-the-national-flock-a-never-ending-story (Accessed 22 August 2021)

Animal Welfare Indicators project — Castration of lambs less than a week of age – video. Animal Welfare Indicators Project. www.youtube.com/watch?v=XvKFGSu9bRE (Accessed 22 August 2021)

typically lasts for around two hours — Goddard, P. Sheep. In *Management and Welfare of Farm Animals – The UFAW Farm Handbook*, p. 245. Wiley-Blackwell, 2011

persist for more than 48 hours — Mainau E, Temple D, Llonch P et al. *Welfare Implications of Tail Docking and Castration in Sheep*. Farm Animal Welfare Education Centre, 2017

more attentive to their lambs — Hild S, Clark CCA, Dwyer CM et al. Ewes are more attentive to their offspring experiencing pain but not stress. *Applied Animal Behaviour Science* 132:3–4 (2011), 114–20. doi.org/10.1016/j.applanim.2011.04.003

Several million lambs are castrated — Report on the Implications of Castration and Tail Docking for the Welfare of Lambs. Farm Animal Welfare Council. Department for Environment, Food and Rural Affairs, 2008

no evidence to support the suggestion — IBID

farmland birds having declined more severely — The State of Nature 2019. Hayhow DB, Eaton MA, Stanbury AJ et al. The State of Nature partnership, 2019

As the UK nations' Sheep Welfare Codes – e.g. Code of Recommendations for the Welfare of Livestock: Sheep. Department for Environment, Food and Rural Affairs

the British Veterinary Association and the UK's Sheep Veterinary Society — Position on Sheep Castration, Tail Docking and Pain Management. British Veterinary Association and Sheep Veterinary Society, 2020. https://www.bva.co.uk/media/3364/sheep-castration-tail-docking-and-pain-management-final.pdf (Accessed 22 August 2021)

licensed for use in sheep in Canada and Australia — IBID

Growing numbers of farmers are taking — Gascoigne E, Mouland C and Lovatt F. Considering the 3Rs for castration and tail docking in sheep. *In Practice* 43 (2021), 152–62. doi.org/10.1002/inpr.29

Chapter 10 — Hummingbirds and horses

The UK's Links Group — www.thelinksgroup.org.uk/ (Accessed 23 August 2021)

It is well known that — Recognising Abuse in Animals and Humans: Comprehensive Guidance for the Veterinary Team. Animal Welfare Foundation and The Links Group, 2016. https://www.animalwelfarefoundation.org.uk/wp-content/uploads/2017/12/20160415-AWF-Recognising-abuse-in-animals-and-humans-v10-web.pdf (Accessed 23 August 2021)

estimated 60 million or so horses — FAOSTAT, 2014

used for human recreation or sport — Waran N (ed.). *The Welfare of Horses*. Springer, 2007

Gingering — Heird J. Abusive treatment and subsequent policy development within various breeds of show horses in the USA. In McIlwraith CW and Rollin BE (eds) *Equine Welfare,* Wiley-Blackwell, 2011

Tail nicking — Welfare implications of horse tail modifications. American Veterinary Medical Association, 2012. https://www.avma.org/resources-tools/literature-reviews/welfare-implications-horse-tail-modifications (Accessed 23 August 2021)

worn most of the time — Hepworth-Warren K. The truth about tail blocks. *Equus,* 2021. https://equusmagazine.com/horse-world/tail-blocks-truth (Accessed 23 August 2021)

practice called soring — Heird J. *Abusive treatment and subsequent policy development within various breeds of show horses in the USA.* In: McIlwraith CW and Rollin BE (eds) *Equine Welfare,* Wiley-Blackwell, 2011

Humane Society US YouTube video — Tennessee Walking Horse Investigation Exposes Cruelty. Humane Society US, 2012. www.youtube.com/watch?v=gxVlxT_x-f0 (Accessed 23 August 2021)

Inhumane treatment has become — Heird J. Abusive treatment and subsequent policy development within various breeds of show horses in the USA. In McIlwraith CW and Rollin BE (eds) *Equine Welfare.* Wiley-Blackwell, 2011

American Veterinary Medical Association Issue Brief. https://www.avma.org/sites/default/files/2019-10/PAST-Act-IB-8-2-2019.pdf (Accessed 23 August 2021)

Humane Society Veterinary Medical Association — The painful truth of horse soring. Humane Society Veterinary Medical Association. 2012. https://www.hsvma.org/horse_soring#.YSQAzbBKiM- (Accessed 23 August 2021)

are lobbying — Prevent All Soring Tactics (PAST) Act H.R. 693/S. 1007

the alteration of the tail — Position on tail alteration in horses

AAEP also condemned — American Association of Equine Practitioners, 2015. https://aaep.org/position-tail-alteration-horses (Accessed 23 August 2021)

'alarmingly widespread' — Hepworth-Warren K. The truth about tail blocks. *Equus,* 2021. https://equusmagazine.com/horse-world/tail-blocks-truth (Accessed 23 August 2021)

naturally spend up to 16 hours — Goodwin D. Horse behaviour: Evolution, Domestication and Feralisation. In Waran N (ed.). *The Welfare of Horses*. Springer, 2007

over a third of pleasure horses — Sykes BW, Hewetson M, Hepburn RJ et al. European College of Equine Internal Medicine Consensus Statement – Equine

Gastric Ulcer Syndrome in Adult Horses. *Journal of Veterinary Internal Medicine* 29:5 (2015), 1288–99. doi: 10.1111/jvim.13578

five grades of ulcer severity — IBID

also be linked to stressors — e.g. McClure SR. *Equine Gastric Ulcers: Special Care and Nutrition.* American Association of Equine Practitioners, 2016. https://aaep. org/horsehealth/equine-gastric-ulcers-special-care-and-nutrition (Accessed 23 August 2021)

nearly doubles during the competitive period — Sykes BW, Hewetson M, Hepburn et al. European College of Equine Internal Medicine Consensus Statement – Equine gastric ulcer syndrome in adult horses. *Journal of Veterinary Internal Medicine* 29:5 (2015), 1288–99. doi: 10.1111/jvim.13578

'distressingly high prevalence' — Roberts C. Prevalence of equine gastric ulcers and its prevention. *Veterinary Times,* 2008

'often a man-made disease' — e.g. McClure SR. *Equine Gastric Ulcers: Special Care and Nutrition.* American Association of Equine Practitioners, 2016. https://aaep. org/horsehealth/equine-gastric-ulcers-special-care-and-nutrition (Accessed 23 August 2021)

if only powered by grass — Davidson N and Harris P. Nutrition and welfare. In Waran, N (ed.). *The Welfare of Horses.* Springer, 2007

futile therapeutic recommendations — Roberts C. Prevalence of equine gastric ulcers and its prevention. *Veterinary Times,* 2008

The governing body of equestrian activities — Campbell MLH. *Animals, Ethics and Us.* 5M Publishing, 2019

Crib biting has been reported — Waters AJ, Nicol CJ and French NP. Factors influencing the development of stereotypic and redirected behaviours in young horses: findings of a four year prospective epidemiological study. *Equine Veterinary Journal* 34:6 (2002), 572–9. doi: 10.2746/042516402776180241

from 15 to 65 per cent of their time — Wickens CL and Heleski CR. Crib-biting behavior in horses: A review. *Applied Animal Behaviour Science* 128:1–4 (2010), 1–9. doi: 10.1016/j.applanim.2010.07.002

Using endoscopy to examine — Nicol CJ, Davidson HP, Harris PA et al. Study of crib-biting and gastric inflammation and ulceration in young horses. *Veterinary Record* 151:22 (2002), 658–62. doi: 10.1136/vr.151.22.658

subsequent researchers have concluded — Daniels SP, Scott L, De Lavis I et al. Crib biting and equine gastric ulceration syndrome: do horses that display oral stereotypies have altered gastric anatomy and physiology? *Journal of Veterinary Behavior* 30 (2018), 110–13. 10.1016/j.jveb.2018.12.010

Stereotypies have traditionally been called 'vices' — e.g. Nicol C. Understanding equine stereotypies. *Equine Veterinary Journal Supplement* 28 (1999), 20–5

especially the feeding of low-fibre — Cooper J. Stereotypic behaviour in the stabled horse: causes, effects and prevention without compromising horse welfare. In Waran N (ed.). *The Welfare of Horses*. Springer, 2007

have found nearly a fifth — e.g. Dalla Costa E, Dai F, Lebelt D et al. Initial outcomes of a harmonized approach to collect welfare data in sport and leisure horses. *Animal* 11:2 (2017), 254–60. doi.org/10.1017/S1751731116001452

spend significant proportions of their time caged — Wylie CE, Ireland JL, Collins SN et al. Demographics and management practices of horses and ponies in Great Britain: A cross-sectional study. *Research in Veterinary Science* 95:2 (2013), 410–17. doi.org/10.1016/j.rvsc.2013.05.004. Cited in: Rioja-Lang FC, Connor M, Bacon H et al. Determining a welfare prioritization for horses using a delphi method. *Animals* 10:4 (2020), 647. doi.org/10.3390/ani10040647

no scientific evidence supports this — Wickens CL and Heleski CR. Crib-biting behavior in horses: A review. *Applied Animal Behaviour Science* 128:1–4 (2010), 1–9. doi: 10.1016/j.applanim.2010.07.002

The effect in all cases of physical prevention (1) — IBID

The effect in all cases of physical prevention (2) — Sarrafchi A and Blokhuis HJ. Equine stereotypic behaviors: Causation, occurrence, and prevention. *Journal of Veterinary Behavior* 8:5 (2013), 386–94. doi.org/10.1016/j.jveb.2013.04.068

most commonly triggered — Couëtil L, Cardwell J, Gerber V et al. Inflammatory airway disease of horses—Revised consensus statement. *Journal of Veterinary Internal Medicine* 30 (2016), 503–15. doi.org/10.1111/jvim.13824

a disease 'primarily of domestication' — Mazan RM. Lower airway disease in the athletic horse. *Veterinary Clinics: Equine Practice* 34 (2018), 443–60

one of the most common causes of death — What is colic? University of Liverpool Equine Hospital. https://www.liverpool.ac.uk/equine/common-conditions/colic/what-is-colic/ (Accessed 25 August 2021)

350 colic cases that are seen — Surgery and postoperative care. University of Liverpool Equine Hospital. https://www.liverpool.ac.uk/equine/common-conditions/colic/colic-surgery/ (Accessed 25 August 2021)

'Sufficient access to pasture' — Scantlebury CE, Archer DC, Proudman CJ et al. Risk factors for recurrent colic in UK general equine practice. *Equine Veterinary Journal* 47 (2015), 202–6. doi.org/10.1111/evj.12276

horses displaying crib biting, wind sucking — IBID

In a scientific review paper — Archer DC and Proudman CJ. Epidemiological clues to preventing colic. *Veterinary Journal* 172 (2006), 29–39. 10.1016/j.tvjl.2005.04.002

online BBC video — Horses dance to Phil Collins in Olympics dressage. www.bbc.co.uk/sport/av/olympics/19196356 (Accessed 25 August 2021)

81 per cent of horse owners thought — Bradshaw JWS and Casey R. Anthropomorphism and anthropocentrism as influences in the quality of life of companion animals. *Animal Welfare* 16:S1 (2007), 149–54

stabled for 64–91 per cent of their time — Walters JM, Parkin T, Snart HA et al. Current management and training practices for UK dressage horses. *Comparative Exercise Physiology* 5 (2008), 73–83. 10.1017/S1478061508017040

may not be well supported by research — Hartmann E, Søndergaard E and Keeling L. Keeping horses in groups: A review. *Applied Animal Behaviour Science*, 2012, p. 136. 10.1016/j.applanim.2011.10.004.

Leading equine veterinarian Dr Midge Leitch — Leitch M. Welfare in the discipline of dressage. In McIlwraith CW and Rollin BE (eds) *Equine Welfare*. Wiley-Blackwell, 2011

a separate survey found that a third — McGreevy PD, French NP and Nicol CJ. The prevalence of abnormal behaviours in dressage, eventing and endurance horses in relation to stabling. *Veterinary Record* 137:2 (1995), 36–7. doi: 10.1136/vr.137.2.36

found to become more optimistic — Löckener S, Reese S, Erhard M et al. Pasturing in herds after housing in horseboxes induces a positive cognitive bias in horses. *Journal of Veterinary Behavior* 11 (2016), 50–5. doi.org/10.1016/j.jveb.2015.11.005

Just under a third of horses and ponies — Robin CA, Ireland JL, Wylie CE et al. Prevalence of and risk factors for equine obesity in Great Britain. *Equine Veterinary Journal* 47 (2015), 196–201. doi.org/10.1111/evj.12275

reduced quality of life — Managing a good doer. World Horse Welfare. www.worldhorsewelfare.org/advice/management/managing-a-good-doer (Accessed 25 August 2021)

from the British Equine Veterinary Association — Equine obesity. British Equine Veterinary Association. www.beva.org.uk/Guidance-and-Resources/Routine-Healthcare/Equine-Obesity (Accessed 25 August 2021)

Sixty-six horses are reported to have died — The Grand National Meeting's horse deaths. Animal Aid. www.animalaid.org.uk/the-issues/our-campaigns/horse-racing/ban-the-grand-national/the-grand-national-meetings-horse-deaths/ (Accessed 25 August 2021)

and the high-profile Cheltenham Festival — Cheltenham Festival fatalities. Animal Aid. www.animalaid.org.uk/the-issues/our-campaigns/horse-racing/the-cheltenham-festival/cheltenham-festival-fatalities/ (Accessed 25 August 2021)

848 horses died — Making horseracing safer. British Horseracing Authority. www.britishhorseracing.com/regulation/making-horseracing-safer/ (Accessed 25 August 2021)

The risk of horse fatalities in British jump racing — How safe is horseracing? Jump racing. British Horseracing Authority. https://www.britishhorseracing.com/regulation/making-horseracing-safer/ (Accessed 25 August 2021) *the figure for flat racing* — IBID

a spokesperson for Aintree Racecourse suggesting — Who, what, why: How dangerous is the Grand National? BBC News, 11 April 2011. www.bbc.co.uk/news/magazine-13034474 (Accessed 25 August 2021)

A top trainer also drew a comparison — IBID

a leading Irish trainer made headlines — Gordon Elliott: Irish trainer banned for 12 months for dead horse photo. 2021. BBC Sport. https://www.bbc.co.uk/sport/horse-racing/56290362.amp (Accessed 25 August 2021)

In 2022, a survey by — Public Attitudes on the Use of Horses in Sport: Survey Report (November 2022). Equine Ethics and Wellbeing Commission. Fédération Equestre Internationale (FEI)

The Commission's international survey — Opinions of Equestrian Stakeholders on the use of Horses in Sport: Survey Report (November 2022). Equine Ethics and Wellbeing Commission. Fédération Equestre Internationale (FEI)

For horses, social contact — Krueger K, Esch L, Farmer K et al. Basic Needs in Horses? – A literature review. *Animals* 11:6 (2021), 1798. doi.org/10.3390/ani11061798

2021 BBC Panorama documentary — *The Dark Side of Horse Racing*. BBC Panorama, 2021. www.bbc.co.uk/programmes/m000y2xm (Accessed 25 August 2021)

former jockey, Richard Pitman — Is horse racing too dangerous? *The Guardian*, 13 April 2012. www.theguardian.com/commentisfree/2012/apr/13/grand-national-horse-racing-dangerous (Accessed 25 August 2021)

asserted that horses enjoy racing — IBID

Twenty-five horses are reported to have died — Omak 'Suicide Race' 2018: more dead horses & 'kill the messenger'. *Animals* 14 Sept 2018, 24–7. www.animals24-7.org/2018/09/14/omak-suicide-race-2018-more-dead-horses-kill-the-messenger/ (Accessed 28 August 2021)

5.77 million attendances at 1,500 fixtures — *A Life Well Lived: A New Strategic Plan for the Welfare of Horses Bred for Racing, 2020–2024*. Horse Welfare Board, 2020

Horse Welfare Board published a strategy — IBID

actively promoting the Three Fs — e.g. Calls to rethink turnout measures for horses to benefit their welfare. *Horse and Hound*, 3 August 2020. https://www.horseandhound.co.uk/plus/news-plus/turnout-key-for-horse-welfare-721054 (Accessed 28 August 2021)

EU Animal Welfare Platform's good practice guide — *Guide to Good Animal Welfare Practice for the Keeping, Care, Training and Use of Horses*. EU Platform on Animal Welfare, 2019

In 2022, the Pony Club Australia — Horse Welfare Policy. Pony Club Australia. 2022. https://ponyclubaustralia.com.au/wp-content/uploads/2020/06/PCA-Horse-Welfare-Policy-WEB.pdf (Accessed 2nd March 2023)

Happy Horses section of her website — Happy Horses. www.rebeccacurtis.co.uk (Accessed 28 August 2021)

Chapter 11 — Our animal companions

resilient to the stressful effects of bereavement — Akiyama H, Holtzman JM and Britz WE. Pet-ownership and health status during bereavement. *Journal of Death and Dying* 17 (1987), 187–93

as Serpell points out — Serpell, J. *In The Company of Animals – A Study of Human-Animal Relationships* Canto, 1996

'pandemic puppies' — Packer RMA, Brand CL, Belshaw Z et al. Pandemic Puppies: Characterising motivations and behaviours of UK owners who purchased puppies during the 2020 COVID-19 pandemic. *Animals* 11:9 (2021), 2500. doi.org/10.3390/ani11092500

around 40 per cent of all dogs in the UK — 2018 PDSA Animal Wellbeing (PAW) *Report*. People's Dispensary for Sick Animals (PDSA), 2018. www.pdsa.org.uk/media/4371/paw-2018-full-web-ready.pdf (Accessed 28 August 2021)

estimated fifth of pet dogs — E.g. see references in Salonen M, Sulkama S, Mikkola S et al. Prevalence, comorbidity, and breed differences in canine anxiety in 13,700 Finnish pet dogs. *Scientific Reports* 10 (2020), 2962. doi.org/10.1038/s41598-020-59837-z

The PDSA Animal Wellbeing Report — 2020 PDSA Animal Wellbeing (PAW) *Report*. People's Dispensary for Sick Animals (PDSA), 2020. www.pdsa.org.uk/media/10540/pdsa-paw-report-2020.pdf (Accessed 28 August 2021)

amongst those most likely to be relinquished — Puurunen J, Hakanen E, Salonen MK et al. Inadequate socialisation, inactivity, and urban living environment are associated with social fearfulness in pet dogs. *Scientific Reports* 10 (2020), 3527. doi.org/10.1038/s41598-020-60546-w

Between 2015 and 2018, 23,078 people — Be dog safe, warns surgeon as NHS figures show an increase in hospital admissions for dog bites; averaging at nearly 8000 a year. Royal College of Surgeons of England, 6 June 2019. https://www.rcseng.ac.uk/news-and-events/media-centre/press-releases/be-dog-safe/ (Accessed 5 September 2021)

Researchers at the UK's Royal Veterinary College — Boyd C, Jarvis S, McGreevy P et al. Mortality resulting from undesirable behaviours in dogs aged under three years attending primary-care veterinary practices in England. *Animal Welfare* 27 (2018), 251–62. 10.7120/09627286.27.3.251

this places a significant emotional toll — e.g. 98% of vets asked to euthanise healthy pets – survey. Politics Home, 2016. https://www.politicshome.com/members/article/98-of-vets-asked-to-euthanise-healthy-pets-survey (Accessed 29 August 2021)

See also Batchelor CE and McKeegan DE. Survey of the frequency and perceived stressfulness of ethical dilemmas encountered in UK veterinary practice. *Veterinary Record* 170:1 (2012), 19. doi: 10.1136/vr.100262

Professor John Bradshaw describes — Bradshaw J. *In Defence of Dogs: Why Dogs Need Our Understanding.* Allen Lane, 2011

at best, meaningless and, at worst, inhumane — (1) Bradshaw JWS, Emily J Blackwell EJ and Casey RA. Dominance in domestic dogs—useful construct or bad habit? *Journal of Veterinary Behavior* 4:3 (2009), 135–44. doi.org/10.1016/j.jveb.2008.08.004

— (2) Wynne CDL. The indispensable dog. *Frontiers in Psychology* 12 (2021), 2730—10.3389/fpsyg.2021.656529

around a third are also susceptible — Noori Z, Moosavian HR, Esmaeilzadeh H et al. Prevalence of polycystic kidney disease in Persian and Persian related-cats referred to Small Animal Hospital, University of Tehran, Iran. *Iranian Journal of Veterinary Research* 20:2 (2019), 151–54

unable to breathe freely — O'Neill DG, Skipper AM, Kadhim J et al. Disorders of Bulldogs under primary veterinary care in the UK in 2013. *PLoS ONE* 14:6 (2019), e0217928. doi.org/10.1371/journal.pone.0217928

recurring skin infections and eye ulcers — IBID

unable to give birth without requiring — (1) Evans KM and Adams VJ. Proportion of litters of purebred dogs born by caesarean section. *Journal of Small Animal Practice* 51 (2010), 113–18. doi.org/10.1111/j.1748-5827.2009.00902.x

— (2) O'Neill DG, O'Sullivan AM, Manson EA et al. Canine dystocia in 50 UK first-opinion emergency-care veterinary practices: prevalence and risk factors. *Veterinary Record*, 2017, p. 181. doi: 10.1136/vr.104108

Genetic Welfare Problems website — Genetic welfare problems of companion animals – English Bulldog – Brachycephalic Airway Obstruction Syndrome. www.ufaw.org.uk/dogs/english-bulldog-brachycephalic-airway-obstruction-syndrome-baos (Accessed 30 August 2021)

soared in popularity in recent years — Consensus on advice for anyone thinking of purchasing a brachycephalic dog. UK Brachycephalic Working Group, 2021. www.ukbwg.org.uk/wp-content/uploads/2021/03/210321-BWG-Consensus-Stop-and-think-before-buying-a-flat-faced-dog.pdf (Accessed 30 August 2021)

The UK's Brachycephalic Working Group — www.ukbwg.org.uk (Accessed 30 August 2021)

The group also supports the appropriate use of legislation — Position Statement on Legislation relating to Brachycephalic Dogs in the UK. UK Brachycephalic Working Group, 2021. www.ukbwg.org.uk/wp-content/uploads/2021/06/Brachycephalic-Working-Group-Legislation-Position-Statement-210624.pdf (Accessed 30 August 2021)

Animal welfare laws applying in England since 2018, and Scotland since 2021 —

The Animal Welfare (Licensing of Activities Involving Animals) (England) Regulations 2018

The Animal Welfare (Licensing of Activities Involving Animals) (Scotland) Regulations 2021

In a Royal Veterinary College study — Packer R, Hendricks A and Burn C. Do dog owners perceive the clinical signs related to conformational inherited disorders as 'normal' for the breed? A potential constraint to improving canine welfare. *Animal Welfare* 21 (2012), 81. doi:10.7120/096272812X13345905673809

Over half of cat owners with an overweight cat — 2012 PDSA Animal Wellbeing (PAW) Report. People's Dispensary for Sick Animals (PDSA), 2012. www.pdsa.org.uk/media/2586/pdsa_animal_wellbeing_report_2012.pdf (Accessed 30 August 2021)

some 6 million pet dogs, cats and rabbits — 2016 PDSA Animal Wellbeing (PAW) Report. People's Dispensary for Sick Animals (PDSA). 2016. www.pdsa.org.uk/media/2628/pdsa-paw-report-2016-view-online.pdf (Accessed 31 August 2021)

around four out of every ten pets — German A. Obesity in companion animals. *In Practice* 32 (2010), 42–50. doi.org/10.1136/inp.b5665

their reduced quality of life — German AJ, Holden SL, Wiseman-Orr ML et al. Quality of life is reduced in obese dogs but improves after successful weight loss. *Veterinary Journal* 192:3 (2012), 428–34. doi.org/10.1016/j.tvjl.2011.09.015

just under half report that feeding treats — 2016 PDSA Animal Wellbeing (PAW) Report. People's Dispensary for Sick Animals (PDSA), 2016. www.pdsa.org.uk/media/2628/pdsa-paw-report-2016-view-online.pdf (Accessed 31 August 2021)

dying two years prematurely — Kealy RD, Lawler DF, Ballam JM et al. Effects of diet restriction on life span and age-related changes in dogs. *Journal of the American Veterinary Medical Association* 220 (2002), 1315–20

many prefer not to live with other cats — Code of practice for the welfare of cats. Department for Environment, Food and Rural Affairs, 2017. https://assets.publishing.service.gov.uk/government/uploads/system/uploads/attachment_data/file/697941/pb13332-cop-cats-091204.pdf. (Accessed 31 August 2021)

around four and a half million cats — 2020 PDSA Animal Wellbeing (PAW) Report. People's Dispensary for Sick Animals (PDSA), 2020. www.pdsa.org.uk/media/10540/pdsa-paw-report-2020.pdf (Accessed 31 August 2021)

reporting that their cat lives with — IBID

4 per cent of households with two cats — Wensley S, Betton V, Gosschalk K et al. Driving evidence-based improvements for the UK's 'Stressed. Lonely. Overweight. Bored. Aggressive. Misunderstood...but loved' companion animals. *Veterinary Record* 189 (2021), no-no e7. doi.org/10.1002/vetr.7

half provide one or no water bowls — *2020 PDSA Animal Wellbeing (PAW) Report*. People's Dispensary for Sick Animals (PDSA), 2020. www.pdsa.org.uk/media/10540/pdsa-paw-report-2020.pdf (Accessed 31 August 2021)

harmful to their digestive and dental health — (1) Prebble JL and Meredith AL. Food and water intake and selective feeding in rabbits on four feeding regimes. Journal of *Animal Physiology and Animal Nutrition* 98 (2014), 991–1000. doi. org/10.1111/jpn.12163

— (2) Meredith AL, Prebble JL and Shaw DJ. Impact of diet on incisor growth and attrition and the development of dental disease in pet rabbits. *Journal of Small Animal Practice* 56 (2015), 377–82. doi.org/10.1111/jsap.12346

do not meet their psychological need — Prebble JL, Langford FM, Shaw DJ et al. The effect of four different feeding regimes on rabbit behaviour. *Applied Animal Behaviour Science* 169 (2015), 86–92. doi.org/10.1016/j.applanim.2015.05.003

If rabbits were fed — The correct way to feed your rabbits and keep their teeth healthy. PDSA, BSAVA, BVA, BVNA, BVZS, RSPCA, RWAF, Wood Green. https://www.pdsa.org.uk/media/6177/feeding-rabbits.pdf (Accessed 31 August 2021)

a fifth of the UK's pet rabbits — *2020 PDSA Animal Wellbeing (PAW) Report*. People's Dispensary for Sick Animals (PDSA), 2020. www.pdsa.org.uk/media/10540/pdsa-paw-report-2020.pdf (Accessed 31 August 2021)

percentage feeding muesli-type food — IBID

In a study of domesticated rabbits — Seaman SC, Waran NK, Mason G et al. Animal economics: assessing the motivation of female laboratory rabbits to reach a platform, social contact and food. *Animal Behaviour* 75:1 (2008), 31–42

doi.org/10.1016/j.anbehav.2006.09.031

48 per cent currently living alone — *2021 PDSA Animal Wellbeing (PAW) Report*. People's Dispensary for Sick Animals (PDSA), 2021. www.pdsa.org.uk/get-involved/our-campaigns/pdsa-animal-wellbeing-report/paw-report-2021/pet-acquisition (Accessed 31 August 2021)

67 per cent living alone in 2011 — *2011 PDSA Animal Wellbeing (PAW) Report*. People's Dispensary for Sick Animals (PDSA), 2011. www.pdsa.org.uk/media/2584/pdsa_animal_wellbeing_report_2011.pdf (Accessed 31 August 2021)

UK veterinary profession's #ItTakesTwo campaign — #ItTakesTwo: Companionship in rabbits is key to their welfare, say vets. British Veterinary Association, British Small Animal Veterinary Association, British Veterinary Zoological Society, 2020.

www.bva.co.uk/news-and-blog/news-article/ittakestwo-companionship-in-rabbits-is-key-to-their-welfare-say-vets/ (Accessed 31 August 2021)

a neutered male with a neutered female — e.g. *Good Practice Code for the Welfare of Rabbits.* All-Party Parliamentary Group for Animal Welfare, 2021. https://apgaw.org/wp-content/uploads/2021/06/Rabbit-CoP-2021-1.pdf (Accessed 31 August 2021)

estimated to affect 10 to 15 per cent — Kubiak, M. Feather plucking in parrots. *In Practice* 37 (2015), 87–95. doi.org/10.1136/inp.h234

cognitive abilities comparable to toddlers — Pepperberg I. Cognitive and Communicative abilities of grey parrots. *Current Directions in Psychological Science* 11 (2002), 83–7. 10.1111/1467-8721.00174

Dr John Chitty, has written — Chitty, J. Feather plucking in psittacine birds 2. Social, environmental and behavioural considerations. *In Practice* 25 (2003), 550–55. doi.org/10.1136/inpract.25.9.550

Dr Rachel Schmid and her colleagues — Schmid R, Doherr MG and Steiger A. The influence of the breeding method on the behaviour of adult African grey parrots (*Psittacus erithacus*). *Applied Animal Behaviour Science* 98:3–4 (2006), 293–307. doi.org/10.1016/j.applanim.2005.09.002

Over half of all households in the UK — *2017 PDSA Animal Wellbeing (PAW) Report.* People's Dispensary for Sick Animals (PDSA), 2017. www.pdsa.org.uk/media/3290/pdsa-paw-report-2017_online-3.pdf (Accessed 31 August 2021)

Some studies suggest — e.g. Paul ES and Serpell JA. Childhood pet keeping and humane attitudes in young adulthood. *Animal Welfare* 2 (1993), 321–37

In 2017, the British Veterinary Association's — Davis N. Mine's a puguccino: pug-themed cafes and events 'irresponsible', say vets. *The Guardian*, 6 October 2017. www.theguardian.com/lifeandstyle/2017/oct/06/mines-a-puguccino-pug-themed-cafes-and-events-irresponsible-say-vets (Accessed 1 September 2021)

pet clothing market is reported to have grown — *Pet Clothing Market Size.* Fortune Business Insights. 2021. https://www.fortunebusinessinsights.com/pet-clothing-market-104419 (Accessed 1 September 2021)

has concluded that many of the UK's pets — Wensley S, Betton V, Gosschalk K et al. Driving evidence-based improvements for the UK's 'Stressed. Lonely. Overweight. Bored. Aggressive. Misunderstood...but loved' companion animals. *Veterinary Record* 189 (2021), no-no e7. doi.org/10.1002/vetr.7

some of Pythagoras' thoughts — Ovid, *The Teachings of Pythagoras.* Republished as pages 367–79 in *Ovid's Metamorphoses* (R. Humphries, translator). Indiana University Press, 1955. Cited in Fraser D. *Understanding Animal Welfare – The Science in its Cultural Context.* Wiley-Blackwell, 2008

the parrot family faces a higher rate of extinction — Olah G, Butchart SHM, Symes A et al. Ecological and socio-economic factors affecting extinction risk in parrots.

Biodiversity and Conservation 25 (2016), 205–23. doi.org/10.1007/s10531-015-1036-z

pre-export mortality rates of 40 to 66 per cent — Mortality rates referenced at: Wensley S. Trade in wild birds. *Veterinary Record* 159:9 (2006), 292. doi:10.1136/vr.159.9.292

published in the Veterinary Times — Tuckey, J. DEFRA should continue any live bird ban. *Veterinary Times*, 20 March 2006

the veterinary profession was calling for the current ban — *Position Statement on the Import of Captive Live Birds.* British Veterinary Association, 2006

adopted by the Federation of Veterinarians of Europe — *Position Statement on the Import of Captive Live Birds*. Federation of Veterinarians of Europe, 2006. https://fve.org/cms/wp-content/uploads/fve_06_001_ban_on_import_wild_birds.pdf (Accessed 1 September 2021)

news came on 11 January 2007 — EU agrees permanent ban on imports of wild-caught birds. *Veterinary Record* 160 (2007), 67–8. doi.org/10.1136/vr.160.3.67

spare around four million wild birds every year — EU ends wild bird imports. *PsittaScene* 19:1 (2007) 3

The philosopher Professsor Bernard Rollin — Rollin, BE. Equine welfare and ethics. In McIlwraith CW and Rollin BE (eds) *Equine Welfare*. Wiley-Blackwell, 2011

A growing percentage of prospective pet owners — *2020 PDSA Animal Wellbeing (PAW) Report.* People's Dispensary for Sick Animals (PDSA), 2020. www.pdsa.org.uk/media/10540/pdsa-paw-report-2020.pdf (Accessed 1 September 2021)

typically offered for free or low-cost — *2018 PDSA Animal Wellbeing (PAW) Report.* People's Dispensary for Sick Animals (PDSA), 2018. www.pdsa.org.uk/media/4371/paw-2018-full-web-ready.pdf (Accessed 1 September 2021)

the Cat Group website — The Kitten Checklist. www.thecatgroup.org.uk (Accessed 1 September 2021)

nearly a quarter of UK pet dog, cat and rabbit owners — *2018 PDSA Animal Wellbeing (PAW) Report.* People's Dispensary for Sick Animals (PDSA), 2018. www.pdsa.org.uk/media/4371/paw-2018-full-web-ready.pdf (Accessed 1 September 2021)

Lucy's Law came into force — Lucy's Law spells the beginning of the end for puppy farming. Department for Environment, Food and Rural Affairs, 2020. www.gov.uk/government/news/lucys-law-spells-the-beginning-of-the-end-for-puppy-farming (Accessed 1 September 2021)

the paradox well described by James Serpell — Serpell, J. *In The Company of Animals – A Study of Human–Animal Relationships*. Canto, 1996

Chapter 12 — The power of one

a million animal and plant species heading towards extinction — Brondizio ES, Settele J et al (eds). Global assessment report on biodiversity and ecosystem services of the Intergovernmental Science-Policy Platform on Biodiversity and Ecosystem Services (IPBES). IPBES, 2019. IPBES secretariat, Bonn, Germany.

one in seven of the world's bird species — International Union for Conservation of Nature (IUCN) Red List of Threatened Species. Summary Statistics. https://www.iucnredlist.org/resources/summary-statistics (Accessed 1 September 2021)

The One Planet Living initiative — What is One Planet Living? www.bioregional.com/one-planet-living (Accessed 1 September 2021)

Or planetary boundaries — Steffen W, Richardson K, Rockstrom J et al. Planetary boundaries: Guiding human development on a changing planet. *Science* 347:6223 (2015), 347–57

As the United Nations says — United Nations Sustainable Development Goals. Goal 12: Ensure sustainable consumption and production patterns. https://unstats.un.org/sdgs/report/2019/goal-12/ (Accessed 1 September 2021)

Dr Kate Rawles has noted — Rawles, K. Environmental ethics and animal welfare: re-forging a necessary alliance. In Dawkins MS and Bonney R (eds). *The Future of Animal Farming*. Blackwell, 2008

The UK government's advisory — *Report on Economics and Farm Animal Welfare*. Farm Animal Welfare Committee, 2011

the Biophilia Hypothesis — Wilson, EO. *Biophilia: The Human Bond with Other Species*. Harvard University Press, 1984

space for reflection and psychological restoration — e.g. Fuller R, Irvine K, Devine-Wright P et al. Psychological benefits of greenspace increase with biodiversity. *Biology Letter* 3 (2007), 390–94. 10.1098/rsbl.2007.0149

According to Wilson's collaborator — Kellert SR. The biological basis for human values of nature. In: Kellert SR and Wilson EO (eds). *The Biophilia Hypothesis*. 1st edition, 1983

nearly a quarter of UK front gardens — *Greening Grey Britain*. Royal Horticultural Society (RHS), 2015. www.rhs.org.uk/communities/archive/PDF/Greener-Streets/greening-grey-britain-report.pdf (Accessed 1t September 2021)

strong and consistent evidence — Lovell R and Maxwell S. *Health and the Natural Environment: A Review of Evidence, Policy, Practice and Opportunities for the Future*. Department for Environment, Food and Rural Affairs (DEFRA), 2018

Numerous studies have revealed psychological benefits — IBID

benefits increase with the amount of biodiversity — Fuller R, Irvine K, Devine-Wright P et al. Psychological benefits of greenspace increase with biodiversity. *Biology Letters* 3 (2007), 390–94. 10.1098/rsbl.2007.0149

are those most closely associated with improved health — Lovell R and Maxwell S. *Health and the Natural Environment: A Review of Evidence, Policy, Practice and Opportunities for the Future.* Department for Environment, Food and Rural Affairs (DEFRA), 2018

proportion of children in high-income countries — Oswald TK, Rumbold AR, Kedzior SGE et al. Psychological impacts of 'screen time' and 'green time' for children and adolescents: A systematic scoping review. *PLoS ONE* 15:9 (2020), e0237725. doi.org/10.1371/journal.pone.0237725

A report commissioned by the National Trust — Moss S. *Natural Childhood.* National Trust, 2012

first ever People and Nature Survey for England — *The People and Nature Survey for England.* Natural England. www.gov.uk/government/collections/people-and-nature-survey-for-england (Accessed 1 September 2021)

87% of adults agreed — *The People and Nature Survey for England: Monthly interim indicators for April 2020 (Experimental Statistics).* Natural England, June 2020

83% of children agreed — *The People and Nature Survey for England: Children's Survey (Experimental Statistics).* Natural England, October 2020

public health professionals cautioning — Gray S and Kellas A. Covid-19 has highlighted the inadequate, and unequal, access to high quality green spaces. *The BMJ Opinion*, 3 July 2020. https://blogs.bmj.com/bmj/2020/07/03/covid-19-has-highlighted-the-inadequate-and-unequal-access-to-high-quality-green-spaces/ (Accessed 1 September 2021)

71% of children from ethnic minority backgrounds — *The People and Nature Survey for England: Children's Survey (Experimental Statistics).* Natural England, October 2020

environmental concern was high amongst children — IBID

What Has Nature Ever Done For Us? — Juniper, T. *What Has Nature Ever Done For Us?* Profile Books, 2013

In 2006, Sir Nicholas Stern — Stern N. *Stern Review on the Economics of Climate Change.* HM Treasury, 2006

As the Native American prophecy goes – Speake J (ed). *Oxford Dictionary of Proverbs.* 6th edition; 2015

Professor John McInerney describes — McInerney JP. *Animal Welfare, Economics and Policy.* Report to Department for Environment, Food and Rural Affairs, 2004

organisations such as Population Matters — Population Matters. www.populationmatters.org (Accessed 2 September 2021)

some having predicted a potential doubling — Meat and meat products. Food and Agriculture Organization of the United Nations. http://www.fao.org/ag/againfo/themes/en/meat/home.html (Accessed 2 September 2021) *graze land that could not be used to grow crops* — Garnett, T. Livestock and climate change. In D'Silva J and Webster J (eds). *The Meat Crisis,* 2nd edition. Earthscan, 2017

Around 30 per cent of former rainforest areas — Bernues, A. Animals on the land. In D'Silva J and Webster J (eds). *The Meat Crisis,* 2nd edition. Earthscan, 2017

accounts for an estimated 14.5 per cent — Gerber PJ, Steinfeld H, Henderson B et al. *Tackling Climate Change through Livestock – A Global Assessment of Emissions and Mitigation Opportunities.* Food and Agriculture Organization of the United Nations (FAO), 2013

global animal agriculture can be a significant contributor — e.g. *Policy Position on UK Sustainable Animal Agriculture.* British Veterinary Association, 2019. https://www.bva.co.uk/media/1181/bva-position-on-uk-sustainable-animal-agriculture-full.pdf (Accessed 2 September 2021)

higher level of consumption of red meat — e.g. Zheng Y, Li Y, Satija A et al. Association of changes in red meat consumption with total and cause specific mortality among US women and men: two prospective cohort studies *British Medical Journal* 365 (2019), l2110. doi:10.1136/bmj.l2110

Medical bodies including Public Health England — *A Quick Guide to the Government's Healthy Eating Recommendations.* Public Health England, 2018 https://assets.publishing.service.gov.uk/government/uploads/system/uploads/attachment_data/file/742746/A_quick_guide_to_govt_healthy_eating_update.pdf (Accessed 2 September 2021)

double the optimal amount of processed meat — GBD 2017 Diet Collaborators. Health effects of dietary risks in 195 countries, 1990–2017: a systematic analysis for the Global Burden of Disease Study 2017. *The Lancet* 393 (2019), 1958–72. doi.org/10.1016/S0140-6736(19)30041-8

In the UK, around a third of the population — *National Food Strategy – An Independent Review for Government: The Plan.* 2021

urging health professionals to help their patients — *All-Consuming: Building A Healthier Food System for People and Planet.* UK Health Alliance on Climate Change, 2020

nearly 690 million people are hungry — *The State of Food Security and Nutrition in the World 2020. Transforming Food Systems for Affordable Healthy Diets.* FAO, IFAD, UNICEF, WFP and WHO, 2020. doi.org/10.4060/ca9692en

over 650 million are obese — Obesity and overweight. World Health Organisation. www.who.int/news-room/fact-sheets/detail/obesity-and-overweight (Accessed 2 September 2021)

As Professor Jimmy Bell — What caused the obesity crisis in the West? BBC, 2012. www.bbc.co.uk/news/health-18393391 (Accessed 2 September 2021)

In its 2011 Report — *Report on Economics and Farm Animal Welfare.* Farm Animal Welfare Committee, 2011

In the 1960s, UK households — Cited in *Farm Animal Welfare in Great Britain: Past, Present and Future.* Farm Animal Welfare Council, 2009

Now, around ten per cent is typical — *Family Food 2018/19.* Department for Environment, Food and Rural Affairs, 2020. www.gov.uk/government/statistics/family-food-201819/family-food-201819 (Accessed 2 September 2021)

Among European citizens 59 per cent — *Special Eurobarometer 442 – Attitudes of Europeans towards Animal Welfare.* European Commission, 2016

57 per cent of US citizens — Spain CV, Freund D, Mohan-Gibbons H et al. Are they buying it? United States consumers' changing attitudes toward more humanely raised meat, eggs, and dairy. *Animals* 8:8 (2018), 128. doi:10.3390/ani8080128

Economist Professor Richard Bennett — Bennett R, Kehlbacher A and Balcombe K. A method for the economic valuation of animal welfare benefits using a single welfare score. *Animal Welfare* 21:S1 (2012), 125–130. doi.org/10.7120/096272 812X13345905674006

only 38 per cent felt well informed — Kehlbacher A. Willingness to pay for animal welfare in livestock production. PhD thesis. University of Reading, 2010. Cited in *Report on Economics and Farm Animal Welfare.* Farm Animal Welfare Committee, 2011

Europe-wide, 64 per cent of citizens — *Special Eurobarometer 442 – Attitudes of Europeans towards Animal Welfare.* European Commission, 2016

approximately 75 per cent of emerging infectious diseases — Van Nieuwkoop M and Eloit M. We must invest in pandemic prevention to build an effective global health architecture. World Bank Blog, 12 May 2021. https://blogs.worldbank.org/voices/we-must-invest-pandemic-prevention-build-effective-global-health-architecture (Accessed 2 September 2021)

Recently, both the European Commission — *Farm to Fork Strategy.* European Commission, 2020

and the UK government have — *Action Plan for Animal Welfare.* Department for Environment, Food and Rural Affairs, 2021. www.gov.uk/government/publications/action-plan-for-animal-welfare/action-plan-for-animal-welfare (Accessed 3 September 2021)

the British Veterinary Association has produced — Choose assured products for animal welfare. British Veterinary Association. www.bva.co.uk/take-action/choose-assured-farm-assurance-campaign/ (Accessed 3 September 2021)

UK sales of ethical food and drink — *Food Statistics in Your Pocket: Prices and Expenditure.* Department for Environment, Food and Rural Affairs. www.gov.uk/government/statistics/food-statistics-pocketbook/food-statistics-in-your-pocket-prices-and-expenditure (Accessed 3 September 2021)

'we are only producing what the public wants' — Harrison, R. *Animal Machines.* Vincent Stuart, 1964

reports that the average UK household — *Digest of Waste and Resource Statistics – 2018 edition*. Department for Environment, Food and Rural Affairs, 2018

In 2012, the cost to save — McCarthy DP, Donald PF, Scharlemann JP et al, Wiedenfeld DA, Butchart SH. Financial costs of meeting global biodiversity conservation targets: current spending and unmet needs. *Science* 338:6109 (2012), 946–9. doi: 10.1126/science.1229803

Martin Harper, former Conservation Director — Financing nature – there is now a will and a way. Martin Harper's blog. 2 March 2018.

US sales of pet treats are today — State of the US pet food and treat industry, 2020. Pet Food Processing. www.petfoodprocessing.net/articles/14294-state-of-the-us-pet-food-and-treat-industry-2020 (Accessed 3 September 2021)

having increased by 29 per cent — US sales of pet treats outpace dog/cat food over the last five years. Mintel, 2017. www.mintel.com/press-centre/social-and-lifestyle/us-sales-of-pet-treats-outpace-dogcat-food-over-the-last-five-years (Accessed 3 September 2021)

UK dog treats continued a decade-long — Value of dog treats market in the United Kingdom (UK) from 2007 to 2018. www.statista.com/statistics/469902/dog-treats-sales-value-united-kingdom-uk/ (Accessed 3 September 2021)

attributed to, amongst other factors — e.g. Pet humanisation and gifting boosts spending. Pet Business World. www.petbusinessworld.co.uk/news/feed/pet-humanisation-and-gifting-boosts-spending (Accessed 3 September 2021)

91 per cent of dog owners and 81 per cent of cat owners — *2018 PDSA Animal Wellbeing (PAW) Report*. People's Dispensary for Sick Animals (PDSA), 2018. www.pdsa.org.uk/media/4371/paw-2018-full-web-ready.pdf (Accessed 3 September 2021)

promoted by the British Veterinary Association — *Policy Position on UK Sustainable Animal Agriculture*. British Veterinary Association. 2019. https://www.bva.co.uk/media/1181/bva-position-on-uk-sustainable-animal-agriculture-full.pdf

In the UK, flexitarianism — *Consumer Focus: The Rise of Plant-based Food Products and Implications for Meat and Dairy*. Agriculture and Horticulture Development Board, 2018

Twenty-one per cent of British people — IBID

investors are said to view the market — IBID

in the 2020 Benchmark, 23 companies — Amos N Sullivan R and Williams NR. *The Business Benchmark on Farm Animal Welfare Report*. 2020. www.bbfaw.com/media/1942/bbfaw-report-2020.pdf (Accessed 3 September 2021)

Good Farm Animal Welfare Awards — www.compassioninfoodbusiness.com/awards (Accessed 3 September 2021)

Following lobbying on gestation crates — Shields S, Shapiro P and Rowan A. A decade of progress toward ending the intensive confinement of farm animals in the United States. *Animals* 7:5 (2017), 40. doi:10.3390/ani7050040

limiting meat to two to three times a week — Karl-Heinz E, Haberl H, Krausmann F et al This indicative example is taken from recommendations made in *Eating the Planet: Feeding and fuelling the World Sustainably, Fairly and Humanely – A Scoping Study*. Commissioned by Compassion in World Farming and Friends of the Earth UK. Institute of Social Ecology and PIK Potsdam. Vienna: Social Ecology Working Paper No. 116, 2009

— A later study reported that reducing average meat consumption in the UK to two or three servings a week could prevent 45,000 premature deaths a year and save the NHS £1.2 billion: Scarborough et al (2010). Cited in *Principles for Eating Meat and Dairy More Sustainably: The 'Less and Better' Approach*. Eating Better, 2018

— The later *EAT Lancet planetary health diet* gives recommended meat consumption levels in grams per week: 'Aim to consume no more than 98 grams of red meat (pork, beef or lamb), 203 grams of poultry and 196 grams of fish per week.' Willett W, Rockström J, Loken B et al. Food in the Anthropocene: the EAT-Lancet Commission on healthy diets from sustainable food systems. *Lancet* 393:10170 (2019), 447–92. doi: 10.1016/S0140-6736(18)31788-4

UK gardens cover an area larger — Professor Mark Fellowes, University of Reading. Quoted in: More birds and bees, please! 12 easy, expert ways to rewild your garden. *The Guardian*, 12 May 2020. https://www.theguardian.com/lifeandstyle/2020/may/12/more-birds-and-bees-please-12-easy-expert-ways-to-rewild-your-garden (Accessed 5 September 2021)

Various wildlife charities provide free guides — e.g. Royal Society for the Protection of Birds (RSPB), The Wildlife Trusts, The Royal Horticultural Society (RHS)

puppy contract and puppy information pack — www.puppycontract.org.uk (Accessed 5 September 2021)

kitten checklist — The Kitten Checklist. www.thecatgroup.org.uk (Accessed September 2021)

Animal Behaviour and Training Council — www.abtcouncil.org.uk (Accessed September 2021)

Food for Life Served Here scheme — www.foodforlife.org.uk/about-us/food-for-life-served-here (Accessed 5 September 2021)

Greener Veterinary Practice Checklist — *Greener Veterinary Practice Checklist*. Vet Sustain, British Veterinary Association, British Veterinary Nursing Association, Society of Practising Veterinary Surgeons, 2021. www.vetsustain.org/resources/vet-practice-checklist (Accessed 5 September 2021)

fire-capped kinglet — Derived from the firecrest's scientific name, *Regulus ignicapilla*. Latin: *regulus* = a prince or kinglet, ignis = fire + *capillus* = capped.

Index

B

Acknowledgements

My unreserved thanks go to my agent, Jessica Woollard. From our first meeting onwards she has listened to my ideas, understood what I was hoping to achieve with the book, and championed and supported its journey and my writing. I am forever grateful.

At Octopus, I have been further welcomed, supported and guided by Natalie Bradley and all the team. They expertly improved my words and turned them in to a book, for which I extend my fullest thanks.

Charles Foster gave me invaluable support and mentorship that I will never forget.

I am extremely grateful to the friends and colleagues who reviewed early excerpts of the book; they did not know how much their generous and constructive responses would mean to me. They are: Gareth Arnott, Lucy Asher, Vicki Betton, Andy Butterworth, Ruth Clements, Dan Crossley, Marjanne Descamps, Helena Diffey, Simon Doherty, Jennifer Duncan, Cathy Dwyer, Samantha Gaines, Tara Garnett, Jules Howard, Mark Kennedy, Pippa Mahen, Paul McGreevy, Siobhan Mullan, Keelin O'Driscoll, Annie Rayner, John Remnant, Jade Spence, Claire Weeks, Anna Wilkinson and Julia Wrathall. David Main has provided inspirational animal welfare leadership, as well as support to me, over many years. Similarly, to James Yeates, who introduced the concept of an animal welfare footprint, I pay special thanks for his friendship and discussions.

Some people gave unfaltering support during the book's entire gestation. The thanks to them are not only for their strong, in some cases lifelong, friendship, but for their occasionally asking the simple question, 'how's the book going?' They are: Ben Gilbert, Cathy and Neale Jones and their family, Michael Lancaster, David Mallett, Chris McCaughey, Daria Rybak, Mandy Stone, Sue and Chris Wensley, Keith Wensley and Danielle Fildes. Miranda and Nick Krestovnikoff and their family also belong on this list, but with additional heartfelt thanks for the magical years spent discussing our relations with animals and sharing our enjoyment of the natural world. For this to culminate in Miranda agreeing to write the foreword was very special and hugely appreciated.

Those I studied with at Edinburgh University for a Masters degree in Applied Animal Behaviour and Animal Welfare have provided close, personal encouragement, warm companionship and inspiration through their ongoing animal welfare work. One of them, Fiona Rioja-Lang, tragically died in 2019, having cemented her reputation as a compassionate and esteemed animal welfare scientist. I write these acknowledgements with fond memories of her friendship and recognition of her legacy.

I thank the staff and lecturers at Edinburgh and Liverpool Universities. In particular, Charlotte Nevison and Paula Stockley, who supervised my zebra finch project and determined my career trajectory in so doing. While at Liverpool, I met John and Margaret Cooper who persuaded me, as a veterinary student, that my thoughts and experiences had value and were worth sharing. I also thank all those who provided placements, allowing me to accompany and learn from them as they tended to their animals. I hope I have managed to faithfully convey the welcomes, precious time and formative experiences that they each afforded me.

Prior to university, Carol Hughes fostered my earliest interest in writing and Gordon Hockings taught me the value of independent thought.

Only a fraction of the charities doing invaluable work to improve animal welfare and protect our world are included in my chapters, but I commend those that are included as being worthy of a reader's further interest and/or charitable support. Amongst them are: Animal Welfare Foundation (AWF), Compassion in World Farming (CIWF), Crustacean Compassion, Dogs Trust, Eurogroup for Animals, National Trust, One Kind, People's Dispensary for Sick Animals (PDSA), Royal Society for the Prevention of Cruelty to Animals (RSPCA), Royal Society for the Protection of Birds (RSPB), Universities Federation for Animal Welfare (UFAW), World Horse Welfare and the World Parrot Trust.

I have had the privilege of working with engaging and talented people at several organisations, who are committed to creating a better world for animals. My very many thanks go, in particular, to colleagues at the British Veterinary Association, the Federation of Veterinarians of Europe, PDSA, Vet Sustain and the Commonwealth Veterinary Association.

Finally, and most importantly, I thank my family. David and Jackie McCaughey have provided continuous practical support and encouragement. My parents, Peter and Maureen Wensley, are the original source of all that I now recognise as good or fulfilling in my life. I cannot do justice to Jenny, Willow and Enda Wensley. Despite how passionately I may feel about what is happening to our fellow sentient creatures beyond the bounds of our home, the love behind our front door is what matters most.

About the Author

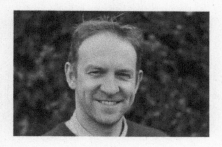

Dr Sean Wensley is Senior Veterinary Surgeon for Animal Welfare and Professional Engagement at the UK veterinary charity, the People's Dispensary for Sick Animals (PDSA). He was President of the British Veterinary Association (BVA) and chaired the Animal Welfare Working Group of the Federation of Veterinarians of Europe (FVE), which represents veterinary organisations from 40 European countries. Sean has contributed to animal welfare and conservation projects around the world and in 2017 he received the inaugural World Veterinary Association (WVA) Global Animal Welfare Award for Europe. In 2023 he received the J.A. Wight Memorial Award from the British Small Animal Veterinary Association (BSAVA) for his outstanding contribution to pet welfare. His media appearances include BBC Breakfast, The One Show, BBC Radio 4 Today and The Big Questions.